# A MOM'S WILL

A Story of Hope and Determination in
Overcoming Will's Mysterious Illness

Jennifer Drake Simmons

Aurora Corialis Publishing

Pittsburgh, PA

Printed in the United States of America

Developmental Editing: Janene Jost

Copy Editing: Allison Hrip, Aurora Corialis Publishing

Illustrations: Will Simmons

Cover Design: Karen Captline, BetterBe Creative

Back Cover Photograph: Details Photography by Melissa Novak

Paperback ISBN: 978-1-958481-08-0

EBook ISBN: 978-1-958481-09-7

# DISCLAIMER

The author is not a medical professional. She makes no claims to diagnose, treat, cure, or prevent any condition or disease. This book is meant to serve as an educational tool for the reader. Please consult with your doctor if you have any questions about starting a new supplement, exercise, therapy, treatment, or herbal regimen.

The advice and strategies found within may not be suitable for every situation. This work is sold with the understanding that neither the author nor the publisher is held responsible for the results accrued from the advice in this book. The content of this book is for informational purposes only and is not intended to diagnose, treat, cure, or prevent any condition or disease. This book is not intended as a substitute for consultation with a licensed practitioner.

Although the publisher and the authors have made every effort to ensure that the information in this book was correct at press time and while this publication is designed to provide accurate information in regard to the subject matter covered, the publisher and the authors assume no responsibility for errors, inaccuracies, omissions, or any other inconsistencies and herein and hereby disclaim any liability to any party for any loss, damage, or disruption caused by errors or omissions, whether such errors or omissions result from negligence, accident, or any other cause.

Use of this book implies your acceptance of these disclaimers.

# PRAISE FOR A MOM'S WILL

"With honesty and vulnerability, *A Mom's Will* opens the doors to Jennifer's heart and invites readers to witness the emotional journey she and her family embarked upon in the face of her son's epilepsy diagnosis and challenges through his childhood.

"Through Jennifer's captivating and raw storytelling, readers are immersed in the rollercoaster of emotions, medical realities, and social implications of raising a child with epilepsy. Moreover, the book highlights the transformative role of nutrition in Will's journey, offering hope and inspiration to other families on a similar path. With every turn of the page, Jennifer's narrative becomes an invaluable resource, revealing the power of resilience, vulnerability, strength, perseverance, and love."

~ Susan Ceklosky
Licensed Sports Nutritionist (LSN) and Certified Weight Loss Coach

———

"Jennifer Simmons is a gift from God. I am so very thankful for her friendship during a dark time in my life. I met Jen through a friend, and I am so grateful for the message to give her a call.

"In 2021, our five year old started having seizures. It was very scary. Thankfully, Jen was always available—a lot of times during the car ride to and from the hospital, we would talk. I would cry. Jen always had reassuring words that everything would be ok. She was always so knowledgeable. We grew to become good friends, and we could see that her son Will and Jonathan are very similar.

"Thanks to Jen and ALL of her help with the Keto diet, our Jonathan celebrated one year seizure-free on June 4, 2023.

"This journey is very hard. I'm blessed my path crossed with Jen. I am so excited for you to read this story and get hope for your journey as well! Congratulations, Jen and her beautiful family!"

~ Lisa Bruce
Mother of five, including a son diagnosed with epilepsy

---

"Mateo's epilepsy diagnosis left us stunned, fearful, anxious, and hopeless—with suffocating anxiety, feeling uneducated and overwhelmed with no support or guidance.

"After a seizure at preschool, a teacher put us in touch with Jen. Our first conversation gave me comfort and hope. Jen spoke my language and helped us navigate through the next several months.

"Jen has been the greatest blessing and biggest supporter throughout our epilepsy journey. Putting our faith in God and having Jen as a support brought us peace and guidance.

"After we had six months of hospital admissions, testing, countless failed medications, and awful behavioral side effects, Jen lead us to keto. The keto diet has kept Mateo out of the ICU and back to life as a five-year-old boy. Mateo will be one year seizure free in July 2022, and we are weaning off our last seizure medication.

"Will's story and his mother's perseverance gave us hope in the darkest of times. We have embraced keto in our lives and Mateo's Doose diagnosis. Mateo now wants to be a keto chef when he grows up."

~Jennifer Tsangaris, MSN, CRNA
Epilepsy mom friend

# DEDICATION

For Will Harrison Simmons—my first born, my inspiration, and my buddy—your strength has amazed me, and I am so proud to be your mom!

For all the families dealing with epilepsy—stay strong and have faith. Hopefully, our story *will* inspire you to keep going. *Where there is a WILL, there is a way,* and we hope you *will* find a way too!

# FOREWORD

By Karen Orr, D.C.

Jen came into my office as someone I would consider a *wounded warrior mom* who needed help to get her body strong so she could keep up the fight for her child and family.

My history with Jen goes back several years before we reconnected in my office in 2013. Looking back, we shared and lived a very similar and parallel path, even though we were more than a few years apart in age. We grew up in the same hometown, went to the same high school, danced in the same dance studio, and moved back to the same area after college, marriage, and having children. We both have two boys with similar personalities and families who share a love for baseball. We quickly connected the dots which immediately set the tone for a very comfortable and positive environment for healing Jen's body—a body that was reacting to some outside stressors, which over the course of several appointments would come to light.

The moment we began talking about Will, I realized Jen was on a mission to give her son the best chance to heal and recover from the health challenges he faced. As a family, they faced these challenges together. She was passionate, open, worried, scared, and tired; yet, she had a quiet strength underneath it all. She had a *will* like no other to figure this out and uncover everything—both traditionally and holistically—to cure Will.

On Jen's journey with Will, and for her family, she became a champion who would not leave any stone unturned. In doing so, she opened up healing opportunities for Will that may have otherwise been overlooked. I believe this greatly enhanced Will's ability to overcome and heal. It wasn't just one treatment, diet, medication, or supplement but a combination of many things Jen would research and implement where and when appropriate. The only constant was her *will*, as a mom, to never, ever give up, in the ever-changing path they were led down.

I was fortunate to be a part of their path. I performed chiropractic adjustments on Will, which helped to calm his nervous system. The real work, however, happened as Jen and I talked tirelessly through topics regarding Will's health history from birth through his entry into the teen years. My role was one of support and understanding as we talked, laughed, cried ... and talked some more. I truly believe God places people where they are meant to be and in the presence of the people they need most at the time. Jen was the strength leading the journey. It was this strength and the support she got from her husband, Brian, that played the ultimate role in Will's ongoing path to healing.

I hope you, the reader, will feel Jen's strength as she tells their story. It truly is one of love, family, and healing.

# TABLE OF CONTENTS

# Chapter 1
# First Seizure

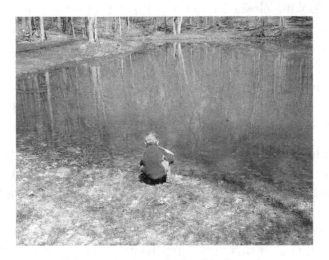

Will (age two) minutes before his first seizure

It was April 2007, a beautiful, sunny spring day, and our family was spending this glorious Saturday out in the woods. Brian's parents, Grandma and G-Daddy, have a wonderful cabin that sits on 100 acres of pristine forest about 50 miles south of Pittsburgh. We'd gone there to enjoy the peace and quiet that nature provides. Little did I know, as we walked amongst the trees, the day would turn out to be anything but peaceful.

Will, who was almost two years old at the time, loved going to the cabin. It's probably his favorite place in the world. He was so excited to get there, go directly to the pond, and feed the fish. Will hopped on the quad with his daddy (Brian) and they headed straight for the water. I followed them down the path to the water with Grandma and G-Daddy. What happened next is forever seared in my memory.

After 30 minutes exploring the pond area, Will just dropped to the ground like a rag doll. At first, I thought he might've fainted, but after looking closer I quickly realized that wasn't the case. His body was lax: like a limp, wet noodle. My heart pounded in my chest as I ran over to see what had happened. The moment Brian picked Will up off the ground, his eyes rolled back in his head, and he began to drool. He was unresponsive, and we were terrified. We were in the middle of the woods with no cell phone reception and no clue as to what was happening to our son.

Brian held tightly onto Will and zoomed up the hill on the quad. They were headed back to the cabin as I desperately tried to reach 911. I wanted to scream at the lack of cell service; there couldn't be a worse possible time. Instead, I began to run—actually sprint—as fast as possible as I followed the roaring sound of the quad engine. It didn't help that I was three months pregnant and still feeling the pains of morning sickness. I couldn't help but think about the stress this was putting on my unborn baby. At the same time, I was consumed with fear of losing my two-year-old child.

Back at the cabin, we finally got through to 911, but were immediately faced with another logistical problem: the cabin doesn't have a street address. It's one of those, *go up the gravel road, turn left at the dirt road, and follow the tree line to the A-frame cabin* kind of directions. While I talked to the dispatcher, Brian tried to wake Will up and was finally successful. Will let out a strangled cry like a newborn entering the world, and I had never been so happy to hear my child cry. He was burning up with a sudden fever and had become extremely lethargic. He just wanted to go to sleep, but we were too frightened to let him.

Twenty minutes later, the ambulance arrived, and Brian, Will, and I jumped in. The EMT asked, "Where to?" and because of proximity, we were forced to select a community hospital to treat our son—a tough choice to make when you can't focus on anything but your sick child. Time was of the essence, and we quickly chose to head to a hospital that was about 20 minutes away. I felt like I was living in a nightmare, or so it seemed at the time. The shrill sound of the ambulance siren, the dazed look on my precious child's face, the fear and panic we all felt, and the persistent worry that the stress of the day could harm our unborn baby was all completely overwhelming.

The emergency room (ER) doctor did a quick exam and suggested that Will had experienced a febrile seizure. Between the quickly spiking fever and the slight ear infection the doctor discovered, he explained that the two symptoms together had likely triggered the seizure. However, as the doctor continued to study Will's chart, he quickly concluded that his symptoms weren't entirely textbook. Will didn't convulse during the seizure; instead, he went rigid and became unresponsive. And so, the testing began.

Our sweet angel was so confused and scared. So were we. Due to the nature of the tests, I wasn't allowed to be by Will's side. The risks of radiation exposure were too great for an expectant mother. It pained me terribly to not be able to be there, not to be able to hold his hand and comfort him in all the ways a mother wants to do. I was beyond relieved to be reunited with Will once the tests were completed. Even more so when his CAT scan had been deemed normal. A couple of hours and a rehydrating IV later, Will perked up. The doctor signed the discharge papers and sent us on our way with instructions to follow up with a neurologist first thing Monday morning. By that time, we were completely exhausted and eager to go home.

The next two weeks were filled with a litany of doctor appointments and a battery of tests and blood samples. Will was really a trooper at first, but it didn't take long for him to figure out what was going on. As soon as we would get close to a doctor's office he would tense up and say, "Go bye-bye." It broke my heart, but I knew we had to get to the bottom of this or at least rule out a couple things. His doctors were checking for brain damage, brain tumors, brain structures, and God only knows what else.

It took two long weeks to get an appointment for the one test we'd hoped would provide some clarity. It was finally time for an MRI. Although we'd become accustomed to all manner of tests by this time, MRIs are different. The subject must remain completely still throughout the procedure. For a two-year-old, that means anesthesia. We were apprehensive about putting Will under, and apparently, he wasn't very keen on the idea either as he couldn't relax for the anesthesiologist. And there I was, feeling helpless to do anything. For the second time, I wasn't allowed to be with him during the test because of my pregnancy. Thankfully, my mom came with us and was able to go with Will in my place. We were blessed that both grandmas were registered nurses, and it seemed like they were going to be put to good use.

It felt like I had waited for hours before I finally saw my mom. She looked distressed as she walked down the hall. Behind her, a nurse wheeled a tiny hospital bed enclosed by cage-like metal bars. I burst into tears at the sight. It didn't help that my pregnancy hormones were raging, but the sight of a two-year-old confined to a hospital crib would be enough to upset any parent.

Will was still out cold and my mom, or Nonny, as her grandchildren named her, was obviously exhausted as well. She'd said that it was probably for the best that I wasn't permitted to go into the room. Things apparently hadn't gone as quickly or smoothly as anticipated because Will was too fidgety for them to conduct the test. What did they expect from a two-year-old during an MRI? So, the team decided to administer an extra dose of sedation medication. In hindsight, I really wish they hadn't.

With the test completed and my child still unconscious, the nurse asked me if I could try to wake him. She warned me he'd be slightly agitated, but *agitated* doesn't even begin to describe it. The poor little guy was a mess. He couldn't walk, let alone hold his head up. He was disoriented and angry, and it was so hard to witness. As they handed me the juice box and snack Will was to finish before leaving—apparently as proof positive that he'd be OK to go home—it dawned on me that when it came to Will, nothing seemed to go as expected.

The sedative that was supposed to wear off in a couple hours, took nearly 24 hours to work out of his system. During those first few hours at home, Will was still unable to walk. He was confused and frustrated, not fully understanding why I was telling him, "You can't walk right now, so just go back to crawling." Fortunately, Will was also exhausted and was able to lie down and take a nap. Much to everyone's chagrin, when he awoke two hours later, he still wasn't able to walk! It was so hard to witness, to try and make sense of it all.

At that point, we needed some answers. I decided to give the nurse a call and ask her some questions. There was a small part of me that felt bad for being a bother but the bigger part of me didn't care. It was my two-year-old son that was suffering; I'm allowed to be a bother! When I got the nurse on the line, I wasn't surprised or particularly pleased with her response. She explained that Will must've had a bad reaction to the anesthesia and suggested that I just keep an eye on him and call back in the morning if he still hadn't improved by then. *Thanks*, I thought sarcastically, *for giving my son a double dose of sedation medication. We appreciate the patience you had waiting for the first dose to kick in. NOT!!* Though we had no proof or prior experience, we believe to this day that Will's extended ordeal was caused by that second, hasty dose of medication.

Thankfully, Will did regain the ability to walk shortly thereafter. And things were somewhat back to normal in the days that followed while we anxiously awaited the MRI results. When the neurologist called to say that they were ready, they asked us to come back to the office to discuss what they'd found. As the neurologist reviewed all the scans, he pointed out some scar tissue in Will's brain and something that he described as delayed myelination. *What?* He might as well have been speaking in a foreign language. I didn't know what that was, but it didn't sound very good. The neurologist went on to explain that the myelin sheath is what covers the nerves in the brain. Will's wasn't fully developed.

Despite the doctor's assurances that this discovery wasn't something to be overly concerned about and that the febrile seizure was likely an isolated event, they also said that Will's seizure was abnormal. Because of that, they decided to prescribe Diastat for Will. Diastat is an anti-seizure medication that is administered anally (Yes, in the bottom!) during a seizure that lasts longer than four minutes. Will needed to have this medication with him at all times. Imagine the conversations I had with family, friends, and teachers who might have Will in their care and could be called upon to administer the Diastat. Not exactly fun.

# CHAPTER 2
## MEET BLAKE RYAN

Will appeared to recover quickly from his ear infection, and the accompanying seizure, bouncing back with the kind of ease that only young children seem to be truly capable of. If only it were as simple for those of us who had witnessed Will's seizure. Every time I closed my eyes I would see his sweet face, with his eyes rolled back, and the drool coming out of his mouth. It was like watching the same awful clip from a frightening movie, playing over and over in a constant loop. I couldn't escape it, couldn't block it out. I know that Brian and his parents felt the same way.

Over time, the fear and anxiety started to fade. The hustle and bustle of our daily lives thankfully diverted our attention. With each passing day, we felt more like our old selves. A little more protective and a lot more observant, but otherwise back to *normal*. We sure were blessed to have two nurses in our family! Even though they are trained and qualified, they were still understandably apprehensive to watch Will on their own—this wasn't just another patient, this was their grandson.

Before I left him in someone else's care, I'd always review the protocol for administering his seizure medication (the one given anally). I could see the trepidation in their eyes, the fear that neither of them voiced but I knew was there all the same. I didn't blame them. How could I? If our situations were reversed, I'd have the same concerns. Heck, I *did* have the same concerns. Honestly, I felt no more ready to counter a sudden seizure than any of the people I'd confidently coached to do so. The difference was I didn't have a choice. They did. But none of my amazing family members or friends ever refused my requests for help and never hesitated to take Will into their care. They just did it with the same fear we had.

Still, we had much to be thankful for in the months that followed. Will was doing well. He started preschool and seemed to enjoy it. A dear family friend was the director, and I felt comfortable leaving him for the few hours he was there each day. He was even placed in a class with a teacher who was also a registered nurse! How lucky were we? She had no problem with the Diastat medication and offered to keep an extra dose at school just in case I ever forgot it. Things were looking up.

Our second child, Blake Ryan, was born on October 26, 2007, and we were all thrilled. Brothers! Will proudly wore his *Big Brother* shirt, and I was so relieved that Blake was here and healthy.

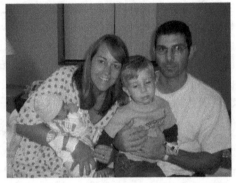

After he was born, I couldn't help but remember the day in the woods when I

Welcome to the world Blake Ryan Simmons

thought I might've put him in jeopardy. When Blake was only four weeks old, I thought my fears might be founded. Blake was born a fussy baby. Constant crying wasn't all that unusual or cause enough for concern, however, a 103° fever was. The fact that Will and Brian had just gotten over a stomach flu made me think that Blake had caught the same bug. Just to be sure, I called the pediatrician. She recommended that I take him to the closest ER. Immediately. *Here we go*, I thought.

When we arrived in the ER, Blake was in danger of becoming dehydrated. I was nursing him regularly at the time, but he couldn't keep anything down. So, the doctor ordered an IV drip. Sounds easy enough, right? Some days it's tough to be an optimist. To be fair, the staff nurses in our local ER probably don't get much opportunity to set up an IV for a four-week-old baby. They had an extremely difficult time trying to find a good place to insert it. It was painful to stand by and watch as they poked and prodded my helpless baby only to fail time and again. I was relieved when they finally decided to call in a pediatric nurse to do the job. At the same time, I felt frustrated and angry that it had taken so long, creating an added and unnecessary toll on my son *and* me. Why wasn't she called in right away? If she had been, we would've known right away that their ER wasn't suited to handle Blake's case. The pediatric nurse took one look at Blake and quickly decided he needed to be taken to Children's Hospital. I could hardly believe that I was about to take *another* ambulance ride with one of my children, but that is exactly what happened. Blake was strapped onto a crib-like gurney, and off we went in the ambulance.

The ride to the hospital went by in a blur. I wasn't quite clear why we'd been sent there. No one even tried to explain. After I registered, my confusion grew as we were placed in a shared room with another family. In and of itself, that would not have been an issue, but the family we were placed with was suffering with an awful stomach bug. One of them was always either on the toilet or vomiting in it. Gross! The doctors really wanted me to continue to try and nurse Blake, so, while sharing a room with a random, nauseated family of four, I attempted to discreetly breastfeed my four-week-old baby. Not a good time. Thankfully, the nurses seemed to realize how uncomfortable we all were and offered to move Blake and I to a private room. I was torn between crying and kissing their feet. Another few hours and I might've done both.

In the comfort and quiet of our own room, my mind began to race. I thought back through my pregnancy and wondered if I'd done something wrong. I was worried about my new baby and wondered just how sick he really might be. Was it something a dose of antibiotics could cure or was it something infinitely worse? The doctor's stream of increasingly specific questions did little to quell my rapidly growing fears. My paranoia went from bad to worse as one evening at Children's Hospital turned into three, and Blake was still feeling sick and listless. His doctors ordered test after test, worried that my baby might be fighting meningitis. The doctors recommended a spinal tap to confirm or deny their suspicions. Though I'd never had a spinal tap myself, I'd heard they were very painful. I couldn't imagine a needle as big as my sweet baby boy being inserted into his tiny, precious back. The doctors didn't want me to accompany Blake to have the spinal tap, and I wasn't convinced I could stand by and watch it, so I hesitantly agreed to stay in our room.

Rather than sit there and stew in my thoughts, I decided to take the opportunity to clean myself up. It had been three full days since we'd arrived unexpectedly at Children's Hospital, and I felt disgusting. I flagged down a passing nurse and all but begged her to point me in the direction of a shower. She pointed me toward the community shower with a fair warning of its dismal condition. At that stage, I had little concern for anything more than the chance to feel clean. So, I borrowed a towel, grabbed some clothes, and marched down the hall. She hadn't been exaggerating—the place was way worse than I'd imagined. Still, desperation can help a person overlook a lot, and that's exactly what I did as I stepped inside the dingy stall and let the stream of welcome water wash over me.

One hour later, I felt refreshed and rejuvenated when they wheeled my little guy back into our room. I sensed from the nurse's odd demeanor that something was amiss. She quickly explained that the doctor tried three times to get the spinal fluid sample but was unsuccessful each time and decided not to try again.

"So, the piercing cries I heard were for not?" I asked, dumbfounded.

"Yes," she replied and then left the room.

Fortunately, I didn't have too much time to wallow in the sea of mixed emotions I was feeling—anger, frustration, guilt—before the doctor came in to offer a diagnosis. He thought it was a virus and wanted to keep us for another night of observation.

*OK*, I thought, *I can do a virus, I guess.* Blake was starting to eat a little more and stay awake a little longer. So, we stayed another night, waited for results from the many samples and tests they'd taken, and drew in deep breaths of relief. Blake was slowly getting better.

My relief at Blake's gradual recovery was tempered by news from back home that everyone there was struggling. Brian and Will had caught the virus the week before and had apparently passed it on to the rest of our family. As soon as one person recovered, another went down, and Will was being passed around to whoever was able to care for him while Blake and I were in the hospital and Brian was at work. I just couldn't wait to get home and see Will and have everyone healthy again. Finally, on the fourth day, we were released and raced home to be reunited as a family. I guess I shouldn't have been surprised when later than night, I was the one that felt sick. My body seemed to fight off the virus while it had to. Maybe the constant adrenaline that flooded my system during our time in the hospital had kept the bug at bay or maybe it was just luck. Who knows? But it was my turn, and I just wanted to be done with it.

What a turn of events! Obviously, with all our attention focused on Blake, Will's seizure had become a distant memory. Finally, with everyone feeling healthy again, we were all hoping for things to go back to normal. No more ambulance rides, no more hospitals, and no more tests. *Please!*

Things did calm down and we returned to life as a typical young family. We just enjoyed each day and appreciated all of the great things that little kids do and say. We were busy raising our two boys and loving every minute of it. We were grateful for the good health that's so often taken for granted, and we happily avoided hospitals and doctor's offices ... for a time.

# CHAPTER 3
# THE GRAND MAL

Will finished his first year of preschool without a hitch and was turning four, which seemed impossible. It really did go by in the blink of an eye. He was doing well and developing on par with other children his age—physically, emotionally, and cognitively. Will was a happy, well-adjusted little boy who loved to run around and play ball with his daddy. He had even started to watch football on TV, specifically the *Yellow Pants,* according to Will. For anyone who might not be familiar with who the *Yellow Pants* are, it's what Will called the Pittsburgh Steelers. He was so excited about watching them play that when his Poppy changed the channel during the commercial break of a pre-season game, Will shouted, "Hey Poppy, put the *Yellow Pants* back on!" It was a wonder to watch Will's personality blossom and grow as he did. We enjoyed getting to know our energetic little boy better and recognizing his likes, dislikes, behaviors, and habits helped us understand what made him tick. We loved him so much.

Summer arrived and with it a whirlwind of play dates in the park, swimming in the pool, and an amazing family vacation to the Outer Banks of North Carolina. We really had a wonderful time enjoying the long, lazy, sun-filled days with our family and friends. One of our last outings of the season was to a minor league baseball game with a big bunch of neighbors and their kids. Being in the ballpark is always a little nostalgic for Brian and me as we spent the better part of a decade in different parks across the country during his professional baseball career. We were excited for the boys to experience all the splendor and spectacle of a minor league game— more known for the oddball contests, eclectic music, plentiful junk food, and fun fan giveaways than for the baseball itself. So, it wasn't much of a surprise that after just one inning, the boys were over the game. Exhausted from the vacation we'd just returned from the day before, the boys faded fast after only a couple of innings. Brian and I decided it was time to cash in our chips and head home.

The next day Will was extremely tired and unusually cranky. I thought, *OK, maybe we just over-did it.* I planned on spending a

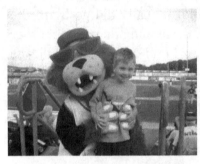

lazy day at home, giving everyone a chance to do nothing but rest and recuperate from our hectic week. Then the phone rang and some of our friends wanted to meet us at the park that afternoon. The boys missed their friends, and I missed mine too. It's wonderful to have good friends with kids the same age as ours. It was going to be a nice day, and the park is a laid-back place to spend some time

Will enjoying an evening at the ballpark the day before his second seizure.

catching up with everyone. So, a couple of hours later, we were off to the park. Will was still acting extra sensitive and seemed oddly clumsy before we left. He had been falling a lot lately, but we chalked it up to him just being tired.

After an hour or two at the park, we returned home. Brian walked into the family room and sat down to play with Will and Blake. I decided that was a good opportunity for me to start dinner. Our kitchen area is openly connected to our family room, so it was easy for Brian and me to chat as the boys played with their toy cars on the floor.

Suddenly, Will jerked up to his knees prompting Brian to ask, "Buddy, what are you doing?" Will didn't respond—couldn't respond—as his eyes rolled back in his head and he fell to the floor, his body thrown into convulsions. Brian yelled, "He's having a seizure!"

I ran from the kitchen and after witnessing the terrifying sight I grabbed his emergency seizure medication. We felt helpless once again as we watched his body violently twitch and jerk. Although it had been two years since his initial seizure, Brian and I had learned a lot in the time between about the *dos* and *don'ts* of assisting someone in the throes of a seizure. After about two seemingly endless minutes, Will's body finally relaxed. He curled up in a ball there on the floor and fell asleep. Rather than dialing 911, this time we simply let him sleep.

We placed him gently on the couch, and I called my mom and my mother in-law. Their shared experiences and insights as registered nurses are always reassuring, particularly in times like this. My mom and dad rushed over right away in case we chose to take Will to the hospital, ready to take care of Blake if needed.

Next, I called Will's neurologist—no answer—the office was closed. So, I dialed the neurologist on call, hoping that one of the doctors who had seen Will before would pick up the phone, but that wasn't the case. I described the seizure and discussed Will's history with the neurologist and was told to just keep an eye on him and bring him in if anything seemed "strange." Well, a lot seemed "strange" to us! What was happening to sweet Will? Why did he have another seizure? How did he go from rolling cars on the carpet with his brother and dad one minute to shaking uncontrollably the next?

This time his seizure was what would be considered a textbook grand mal (or tonic-clonic) seizure. To be honest, I wasn't sure if that was a good thing or a bad thing. It was just so much to take in and sort through. We checked his temperature, secretly hoping he might have a fever and thinking that a sudden spike might indicate that he had had another febrile seizure. Not that a febrile seizure was good by any means—no seizure is good—but there's something comforting about knowing the potential cause behind a seizure: a valid, explainable medical cause. Febrile seizures occur when a child's temperature rises rapidly, usually to 102° or higher, according to the Centers for Disease Control and Prevention website.[1]

Much to our relief, Will woke up about 35 minutes later. I was so happy to see his little face and the usual light of recognition and awareness gleaming in his bright blue eyes. It was as if he had just awakened from a regular, run-of-the-mill nap, stretching and yawning like nothing happened before he'd fallen asleep. I was so relieved, I couldn't stop the stream of tears that began to run down my cheeks, so I turned away. I didn't want Will to see that I was upset; I didn't want to frighten or worry my son.

Ever stalwart, Brian picked Will up and asked him a few questions. He asked Will if he remembered playing cars with him and Blake. He answered, "No." Apparently, he had no idea he'd even had a seizure. Thank God. I began to wonder if the seizures he'd experienced looked worse than how they actually felt? He had no memory of the event and was seemingly no worse for the wear. That's what I hoped for anyway; it's what I wanted to believe.

Brian and I went back and forth for a while about whether to take him to the hospital. Neither of us wanted to submit our four-year-old to more testing, more needles, more waiting, more stress. So, we opted to keep an eye on him at home with plans to call his neurologist in the morning. I knew I wouldn't get any sleep that night. I was filled with worry, and every time I closed my eyes, I saw his little convulsing body. *Talk about a nightmare!* I decided to just sleep with Will, cuddling close like a protective lioness curled around her cub. In all honesty, it probably comforted me more than him to be by his side. He was exhausted from the seizure and found sleep easily. He did toss and turn quite a bit throughout the night.

---

[1] https://www.cdc.gov/vaccinesafety/concerns/febrile-seizures.html

Whether that was par for the course for him or a lingering side effect of his seizure, I couldn't be sure.

The next morning, I called his neurologist. We hadn't been in touch with him in over a year. Anyone who has been desperate for a doctor's appointment knows the drill. The first available appointment was three months away. *Unacceptable!* My four-year-old just had his second seizure, and I needed answers. Thankfully, the scheduler, who was very sweet and understanding, took time to ask the necessary questions to determine how urgent our situation was. In the end, she decided to send Will for an electroencephalogram (EEG), which is a test that measures the brain's electrical activity. She said that she could fit us in the next day, and we happily took the appointment. The thought was that if the EEG is abnormal, we would be given a neurology appointment sooner. If it was normal, we would have to wait for the original appointment in three months.

So, it was time for another doctor's appointment for Will. Luckily, EEGs can be done in the suburban hospital center, so we didn't have to make the trek downtown—so much less stressful for everyone. He was scheduled for a 40-minute EEG. We were told to be there about 45 minutes early because of the time it would take to place and attach the twenty electrodes required to conduct the test. These small, innocuous sensors could (hopefully) help us better understand the complicated and mysterious story of Will's developing brain. As you might imagine, keeping a four-year-old still for that long was no easy task and the staff felt compelled to put Will in a straitjacket. It was disturbing to see my son confined in that way, but I didn't challenge the process.

The technician was a godsend: a wonderfully nice, professional guy who did so much to put both Will and me at ease with his knowledge and calm demeanor. Once the electrodes were secured into place, all that was left was to watch and wait. Will laid still for the next 40 minutes while the electrodes recorded his brain waves.

During that time, he drifted off to sleep ... and who could blame him? It turned out to be a good thing because it allowed the technicians to look at his brain activity while he slept.

I know that the techs aren't supposed to say anything about how a test is going while in progress, but I couldn't help but ask if he thought everything looked OK. He admitted that he'd seen one thing that looked a little suspicious and recommended that we see the head of the neurology group instead of the doctor we had been seeing to that point. When I explained that there was a three-month waiting period he replied, "Not anymore." He called the scheduler himself and got an appointment for us the following week. At first, I was so grateful. Then it dawned on me why he'd been so eager to bump us up in the schedule; whatever he'd seen on the EEG was out of the ordinary, and that probably meant it wasn't good.

The test might've been over, but the residue from the electrode glue lingered on Will's skin and hair for the next couple days—a visible, sticky reminder of another test endured. That stuff is so hard to get off. I promised Will he would get a surprise after the EEG was over, and he was excited to get his reward! We went across the street to the store, and he picked out a toy monster truck. Luckily, I had a baseball cap for him in my car. That glue really did a number on his blond locks, but Will didn't care about his hair, the EEG, or anything else for that matter; he had a new monster truck, and he was happy.

The next week crawled by as if in slow motion, as time does when waiting for results. Every day I kept replaying the tech's words in my mind. There was something suspicious on Will's EEG. *What was going on in his brain?*

# CHAPTER 4
## TEST TIME

The time had arrived for Will's appointment with the clinical director of neurology. We were more hopeful than ever that we might *finally* get some concrete answers. Maybe his EEG would reveal what was going wrong in his growing brain. We'd been stressed about the appointment in the days leading up to it, and I found myself falling deeper into denial—not wanting to believe or admit that something might be seriously wrong with our son. Upon arrival at the local satellite office, we were greeted by the physician's assistant. She spent quite a bit of time with us, asking tons of questions and taking lots of notes. Apparently satisfied that she'd gathered all the relevant information, she excused herself to go speak with the doctor. I was confused at first, maybe even a little miffed. Were we not even going to meet this guy? Was our case not worthy of the clinical director's time? When I realized she'd been gone for a full 15 minutes, my annoyance turned to alarm. Thankfully, before I had a chance to truly panic, the doctor stepped into the room.

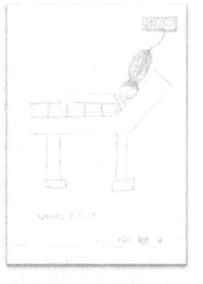

Brian and I both braced ourselves. The doctor was going to explain, at last, what was going on inside Will's brain. The doctor explained that the EEG showed an abnormal activity and that he still wanted more data to get a better idea of what was going on. He ordered a 24-hour EEG and sent us on our way with the number to call to schedule the overnight exam. It was August 6th, and the first available appointment wasn't until September 9th. Waiting over a month was not ideal, but the scheduler assured us that overnight appointments are very hard to get because there aren't many rooms outfitted with the equipment necessary to conduct a 24-hour video EEG test. I guess I should've been grateful that we got in so quick, but at the time, my need for knowledge outweighed my sense of patience and gratitude.

In the interim, school started up again and Will was super excited to get back to his wonderful preschool. And while I was excited for him too, I was also nervous to send him back, still unaware of what was going on in his brain. I set up a meeting with his teacher before classes started to explain what we knew and that we were trying to learn more with his upcoming test. I also confirmed that they would once again agree to administer the Diastat medication that he has to always have with him. I expected his new teacher for the year to be put off a bit when I explained that the medication had to be administered anally and was amazed when she'd said, "My brother has epilepsy so I'm fully aware of what seizures look like and how to handle them." I couldn't believe my ears. What are the chances? She went on to remind me that one of the other teachers was a registered nurse, and she would be happy to store the Diastat medication and administer it if Will ever needed it. My mind was instantly put at ease, and I felt extra confident leaving him with such great people. Once I was sure he was in good hands, it was time to get to the bottom of the madness.

The month flew by faster than expected considering how time crawls when you're awaiting medical tests, news, or results. We were busy with two active little boys, and Will's issues didn't change the fact that we had other things to do and places to be. Blake would soon be turning two years old, and he kept us on our toes. He did his best to keep up with his big brother, and with Will moving a little slower than usual, it was easier for Blake to do. Will had been doing well in his preschool program and had asked to sign up for soccer. So, I found a program and signed him up. Why deprive him of that when we didn't even know what, if anything, was wrong? His very first practice was scheduled for September 9, 2009, the same day he was scheduled to complete the 24-hour EEG.

Soccer practice was scheduled for 5:30 p.m., which I figured would be OK since we weren't supposed to check in to the hospital until 8 p.m. that evening. Will was so excited for his very first soccer practice that he didn't even blink at the fact that I'd been busy packing overnight bags for our trip to Children's Hospital immediately after practice.

In the time following our first visit, the hospital had moved to a new location, and I was actually looking forward to seeing the state-of-the art facility. The hospital was truly impressive. It was obviously designed to welcome and cater to their key clientele—children and their families. It was bright, cheery, playful, and clean, and Will seemed excited to be going for a "sleepover" there, as he put it. I tried to make it seem like an exciting adventure. We packed sticker books, story books, games, special blankets, pillows, and of course Buddy, his favorite stuffed dog. The staff suggested Will dress in button down pajamas so the nurses could easily access the leads that would be placed on his chest to monitor his vitals. Will loved his new pajamas, and I was happy that he did. At the same time, I hated the reason I needed to buy them. Taking your child to the hospital, no matter how nice it is, is always nerve-wracking. The sooner we took the test and went home, the better.

Soccer practice went OK. At least, I think it did. I was so nervous about our pending trip to Children's that I had trouble focusing. Will seemed to have some fun but he continued to act visibly dizzy and disoriented. Every once in a while, I'd even see him just sit down or come off the field without being prompted. We knew something was wrong and it was getting more obvious by the day. It was so strange to comprehend that, just two months ago, he acted like a typical four-year-old boy and now we had no idea what we were dealing with. Sweet Blake was also understandably confused. His big brother was getting all kinds of attention, and we could tell that it was beginning to bother him. No two-year-old could possibly understand, and it wouldn't be fair to expect him to try. For that reason, Brian and I decided it'd be best for him to stay back home with Blake and for me to take Will to the hospital by myself. Besides, we'd been told it was a pretty routine test. What could really go wrong?

That was the last time I went into a test at Children's Hospital with the thought that anything would be routine. As we've already established, Will is not a *by the book* kind of kid, and we were about to be reminded of that ... again.

At first, I thought that things might go better than expected— our EEG tech was awesome! He bounced into our room, full of life, and with a great energy that was refreshing and infectious. He had us follow him to the prep room where he painstakingly placed 20 electrodes on sweet Will's head. Each electrode had to go in a specific place and had to be glued to his head. 45 minutes after he'd started, all the electrodes were finally in place and the room reeked of glue. The 20 wires coming out of Will's head were connected to a little box that was then inserted into a small fanny pack that Will would wear for the next 24 hours. Will was a trooper and stayed very still while the tech did his work. I could sense that it wouldn't be long before the electrodes would become an uncomfortable nuisance. The tech said that he would check in on us throughout the night, make sure everything stayed attached correctly, and ensure that the electrodes contained ample amounts of lotion. Lotion? Yes, lotion. Apparently, the electrodes can burn the skin as they work through the night, so to prevent that from happening, the tech is responsible for keeping them filled with a little lotion. *Great*, I thought. *Just great.*

With electrodes glued firmly in place, we headed back to our room and got set up for the night. Will was supposed to carry on as he would if he were at home with one major difference, he was attached to the bed. The plan was for the team of technicians to monitor his brain activity on the EEG for the next 24 hours while simultaneously watching and recording his physical motions via video camera. They were hoping to capture the kind of abnormal spike they'd seen in the office again. This time though, they'd have a video to go along with the EEG to help them to determine what was going on. I'd been fairly warned that despite their best efforts, sometimes they fail to secure the results they are seeking. The brain is the most complex organ in the human body and

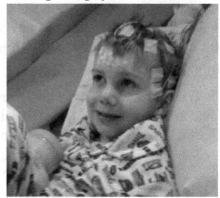

All hooked up with 20 electrodes for a 24-hour EEG

its billions of nerve cells don't always cooperate to give the doctors what they want to see. I thought to myself, *I have only seen two seizures in all his precious four years. There is no way Will would have one now, electrodes affixed and cameras rolling.* One day I'll learn to never say never.

With everything in place and ready to go, Will and I settled in to watch a movie. I climbed up in his hospital bed, removed one of the pads that was supposed to keep him safe, and cuddled close with my little boy. He loved that we were snuggled up together, staying up late to watch a new movie from the hospital's impressive on-demand library. That was a real treat for Will, and all I could do was soak in his excitement. I knew that, soon enough, we would be bombarded by doctors and that Will's electrodes would likely start to itch and annoy him.

When the movie ended, it was time to sleep, and Will didn't fight it. He relaxed on the bed next to me, falling into an easy slumber in no time at all. Not wanting to interfere with the test, I hesitantly crawled out of his bed and tried to get comfortable on the sofa bed in the room. I knew I wouldn't find sleep so easily. Between the various lights and sounds that permeated a busy hospital and the constant stream of questions and thoughts that were racing through my head, it was tough to truly unwind. I couldn't help but wonder what the neurologist in the back room was witnessing. How did Will's brain look? What would tomorrow bring?

The next day arrived with a bang. At 6 a.m., I was awakened by what I thought sounded like labored breathing or choking. I jumped up and was stunned into full consciousness by the sight of my son once again lost in the grip of a grand mal seizure. I was frozen in shock as he convulsed on the bed. The sound of an alarm beeping loudly as he seized rang in my ears as I saw a team of nurses and doctors rush in. They'd obviously seen that he was having a seizure on the EEG and video monitor and quickly came to the rescue. I couldn't believe my eyes as I stood by and watched Will seize for two endless minutes.

The nurses tried to comfort me, but I was an absolute mess. I knew now for sure that there was something seriously wrong with my child, and soon enough, I would know what it was. Will didn't seem to realize what had happened as he drifted off to sleep minutes after the seizure ended. About a half an hour later, the neurologist came in and introduced herself. She started to examine Will and explained to me that the EEG showed more than just the grand mal seizure he'd endured that morning, it also recorded *six* petit mal seizures, one of which had occurred in the last five minutes. My own mind struggled to comprehend what I was hearing: Will had experienced at least seven seizures in the last 24 hours? How was that possible? How many had he had in his life? How many times had he seized in his sleep? I had so many questions, and I felt overwhelmed. I tried to hold myself together, but I simply couldn't. I broke down as the doctor tried to calm my fears.

The neurologist said there was nothing to cry about as she tried to assure me that Will was going to be alright. *Nothing to cry about? Really? He just had at least seven seizures!* She continued to say, "Your son has epilepsy." At that point I began to sob, blindsided by the diagnosis. I really didn't want to cry anymore in front of Will, but I was helpless to hold back the tears. There he was, bravely laying in his hospital bed, confused and scared by my uncontrollable outburst. Thankfully, Brian was on his way to the hospital. In that moment, I needed him to be the calm, logical presence he always is while I struggled to regain my composure.

When Brian arrived, the doctors immediately explained to him what was going on. Although I could see that he was shocked by the news, he maintained the presence of mind to ask some questions about next steps that I was still unable to voice. They informed us that they were going to start Will on a medication called Keppra, an anticonvulsant used to treat seizure disorders. We were told that they wanted us to stay another night so they could insert an IV in Will's arm to get the Keppra in his system fast. Everything felt like it was moving too fast. We went from diagnosis to treatment in the blink of an eye with hardly a moment to consider the course of action. Ever have that feeling like you're watching your own life unfold before your eyes like a spectator at a movie? It was surreal and disorienting, but what choice did we really have? We trusted the neurologists and gave them the go ahead.

It wasn't until the nurse came at Will with the needle and supplies to start the IV that I remembered a foolish promise I'd made to my son before we'd arrived at the hospital: no needles. Will doesn't like needles. What four-year-old does? So, I wasn't surprised at his look of betrayal when he saw what was about to happen. He turned to me and said, "Mom, you promised me, no needles!"

Note to self: never promise your child anything when going to the hospital because you just never know what is around the corner.

I told him all about the overnight EEG and promised him that all the nurse was going to do was put stickers on his head and keep an eye on him. I said verbatim, "No shots, no needles." I lied and he called me out on it at the worst possible moment. I felt terrible. I let him down and there was nothing I could do about it. So, I did the only thing I could do, I crawled back into the hospital bed with him and held him in my arms as the nurse inserted the IV needle and started the medication drip.

While the meds pumped through his veins, Brian and I took some time to learn more about Keppra. It's typically used to treat generalized seizures, and we were told it had minimal side effects. So, as long as Will didn't show signs of an allergic reaction, we'd be discharged in the morning. I was still in shock, but I was also relieved. We finally knew what was happening with Will. We'd been so worried about him and his strange, unpredictable symptoms, but the neurologists had gotten to the bottom of it. Thankfully, Will didn't have any allergic reactions to the medication (I'm not sure my heart could've handled it) so we were finally free to go. Will and I were on our way home with Keppra in hand.

As I tried to settle in back home, I had so much weighing on my mind. One of the things was something that I'd been looking forward to for quite some time. It was Friday morning, and I was supposed to meet six of my girlfriends in Blacksburg, Virginia, for a little college reunion. The trip had been planned six months earlier, and because most of us had little ones, the trip was darn-near impossible to book. The date had finally arrived, and in the weeks leading up to it, I'd been really excited about going back to Virginia Tech (VT) and seeing my girls. But, after three long, stressful days at Children's Hospital, I was completely exhausted and unsure about keeping to my plans. I was emotional and indecisive and needed a little guidance. So, I called Brian on the way home to share my concerns. He always knows what to do and doesn't waver once he's made a decision. He said, "Go! You need to detox after what you've just been through. I think it'd be good for you to see your girlfriends." He assured me that he'd be fine with the boys, taking it easy and spending some quality *guy time* together at home.

My first instinct was to just stay home. Will needed me and above all else, I am a mom. I called the girls to tell them the news that I wouldn't be coming. They were disappointed and so was I. I had planned the trip, made the hotel reservations, and purchased the tickets for the football game that Saturday. Maybe I should go? I really wanted to, but I was conflicted and worried about making a bad choice. Brian was resolute and insisted I go, so the next thing you know, I was packed and headed down the highway. I turned the music up, opened the windows, and tried to leave my worries behind ... look out VT!

I cried most of the drive there, deciding it'd be best to try and get it out of my system before I stepped foot on campus. I didn't want to be the crazy old lady crying in the bar. It felt good—cathartic—just me, my music, and my tears. As I got closer to Blacksburg, the excitement began to set in. I loved that place, and I was about to see my girls ... things were looking up!

I arrived later than the rest of our crew due to the extended hospital visit with Will, so the girls were already out and about. I'd been determined to hold it together, and to put on a brave face, so I checked into the hotel and took a minute to freshen up before I walked across the street to meet them. The moment I saw their familiar faces, the tears just started to pour out. A bunch of warm hugs and one deep breath later, I pulled myself together enough to order a cocktail to quench my thirst and soothe my tattered nerves. It was exactly what I needed.

My friends and I had a great time catching up, laughing, and reminiscing about our time at VT. As the night wore on, the fatigue crept in, and I found myself looking forward to sleeping in the hotel bed as opposed to a couch in a hospital room. I called home to check in and was beyond relieved when Brian promised me that everything was fine. Will was tired, but good. All of them were happy to be home.

The following morning, the girls and I started our day with a trip to the Memorial site commemorating the lives tragically taken on April 16, 2007. Most people remember it as the Virginia Tech Massacre; I choose to think of it as the Virginia Tech Tragedy. The six of us stood around the memorial, holding hands in silence as we remembered that fateful day. Once again, queue the tears. We are all moved by the solemnity of the moment and the sanctity of the place. It turned out to be quite a poignant weekend. As I stood there and read the names of the 32 people that were taken from the world that day, I started to think about how lucky I was to be alive. Those people had been attending class in the very same buildings I had. They weren't doing anything wrong, just going about their day before their lives were ended in an instant. Reflecting on these unfortunate souls helped me to put things in perspective. Life is short, unpredictable, and most of all precious. Yes, Will's condition was concerning and likely to alter our family's life in ways we couldn't yet begin to comprehend, but together we would make it. At the very least, we should feel blessed to have the chance to try.

Minus the tears, we had a great weekend together, and I headed home feeling revived. Everyone had their *stuff* to deal with, and getting together with the girls to commiserate about our unique challenges was a good way to let it all out, get some really good advice, and get a lot of unconditional support. I love those ladies, and though we live in different cities, we will forever share the memories and friendships we forged during our Virginia Tech days. Go Hokies!

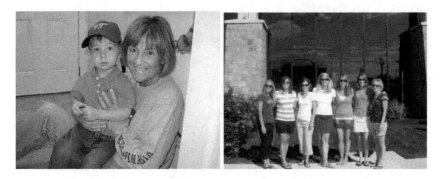

Will and Nonny donning VT gear (left), VT Girls' Reunion (right)

# CHAPTER 5
# INTRODUCTIONS:
# WILL MEET EPILEPSY; EPILEPSY MEET WILL

Will had been on Keppra for about a week when we realized it wasn't going to be the miracle cure we'd hoped. The medication not only failed to prevent the seizures it'd been formulated to stop, but it changed Will's behavior. We no longer recognized our sweet son. He became irritable, angry, and hostile—words I never dreamed of using to describe our easy-going, loveable, little four-year-old before Keppra. Some days I was convinced he was suffering from Tourette syndrome or having some kind of out-of-body experience, like he'd been possessed by some kind of malevolent spirit. He acted meanly toward his baby brother and would lash out at me without warning, throwing fits and objects in his medicine-induced rage.

As if the odd and unwanted changes in Will's behavior weren't bad enough, the number and variety of seizures he experienced each day had literally gone through the roof. The most common type he suffered from is known as drop seizures because the victim loses control of the muscles in the neck, causing the head to drop forward and subsequently hit anything that might be in the way. Sometimes these seizures would knock Will to his knees, prompting me to seriously consider dressing him in a helmet and protective pads. What I really wanted to do was inflate a large bubble and put my little guy inside of it, keeping him safe from the scrapes and bruises that littered his body when he lost control of his brain. Things had quickly spiraled out of control, and I didn't know what to do. We all felt so bad for Will. As a parent, all you want to do is help your child, to take away their fear and pain and make everything better. We started Will on the medication with that end in mind but instead, things only got worse. Wasn't the Keppra supposed to at least suppress his seizures? We were so confused and disappointed. Every day it felt like we were losing more and more of our little boy, and we wanted him back ... badly.

I spent countless hours on the phone with Will's doctors, desperate for ideas on how to make things better. They suggested introducing vitamin B6, indicating that it seemed to help other children who'd exhibited bad behavior while taking Keppra. OK, I figured it was worth a try. What's one more pill-a-day going to hurt, right? Well, I soon learned that it was darn-near impossible to get an adult vitamin down a four-year-old's throat. After a couple tries, I decided to give up and headed to the pharmacy in search of some advice. I loved my pharmacist and the entire staff that worked there. They were knowledgeable and friendly and always willing to help. I was so thankful to have their support when I needed it most. They suggested a pill crusher for the B6, so we decided to give it a try. The pill crusher worked as expected, unfortunately the B6 did not. I pulverized the vitamin and sprinkled it onto Will's applesauce. He didn't seem to notice it and ate it without complaint. Despite the daily vitamin dosage, Will's behavior didn't improve, nor did our hopes that Keppra would be the answer.

After two full, miserable weeks on Keppra, we went back to the neurologist. The medication had done nothing but make Will feel worse, and we were done with it. He was having 30 to 40 seizures a day! He was having different types of seizures with varying intensity, but the sheer volume was insane. The neurologist agreed, and we began the hunt for a new drug. She suggested we try Topamax next and believed it would be a better fit for Will. Due to the incredible frequency of Will's seizures, she also prescribed a drug called Klonopin. Following Will's disastrous results with Keppra, Brian and I were understandably nervous to try these new medications. So, before we had the prescriptions filled, we decided to do some research of our own. Time to go back to the drawing boards.

After doing a preliminary investigation, we weren't particularly psyched about Topamax. The reported side effects were scary, and we were fairly certain our sensitive little boy would experience some of them. The laundry list of potential reactions included everything from kidney stones to memory problems. Despite our reservations, we decided to trust and follow our doctor's recommendation. I mean they should know what's best, right? The second drug the neurologist suggested, Klonopin, is also used to control seizures and calm the brain. It was the latter outcome they hoped to achieve by prescribing this second medication. So, with an inescapable sense of dread, we filled the prescriptions and started the process. As with many potent prescription drugs, anticonvulsants cannot be started or discontinued quickly. The patient has to ramp up and scale down the dosage over a period of time. For Will, that meant he had to scale down on the Keppra while ramping up the Topamax and Klonopin. That schedule made me nervous, and rightfully so.

The same day we filled the Topamax prescription, we had packed the family up for a long weekend in Ann Arbor, Mich. Brian had remained close with a handful of his University of Michigan baseball teammates, and they managed to get together every fall for a football game and a round of golf on campus. We had been looking forward to getting away for the weekend for a long time and decided, despite the uncertainty that surrounded Will's new medication schedule, we would still go on the trip. We sensed it would be an ongoing struggle to figure out Will's meds, but we were determined to do it and determined to keep on living until we did. The more *normal* we all acted, the better Will seemed to do. Focused on a variety of new environments and activities, Will's brain seemed to quiet down a bit as he experienced fewer seizures during our time away.

33

One final factor weighed heavily on our decision to go away when we could've just as easily canceled. It wasn't easy for our youngest son Blake to understand the kinds of challenges his older brother faced every day. All he knew was that Will was acting differently, and so were we. Will was always the center of our attention, even if he didn't want to be. It wasn't fair to Blake, so we took a risk, packed our bags, and hit the road for Michigan.

Luckily, most of Brian's *Good Buddy Guys,* as they call themselves, still lived in Michigan. One family graciously invited us to stay with them and their three sons, which was perfect. Will and Blake were very excited to see their Michigan friends, and so were we! That enthusiasm was tempered though by the prospect of starting Will's new anticonvulsant medications on the road. Over the course of a four-and-a-half-hour drive, Brian and I decided not to start Will on the Topamax that first night

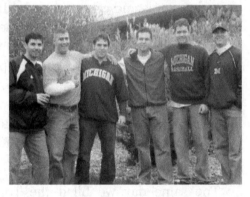

University of Michigan Friends

away. We were anxious and weren't ready to deal with it yet. What difference would waiting one more day make, right? I wish we would have waited forever.

The weekend in Michigan went well. The boys had a blast playing together, and the dads had fun at the football game and golfing. I too had a really nice time. The change of scenery and joy of good company were invigorating and necessary. We decided to start Topamax and prayed it would be *the one.* Keppra was out, Topamax was in, and the watching and waiting began.

After our road trip, we realized the combination of all those drugs swirling in Will's little body began to take its toll. He was struggling, and Brian and I could hardly bear to watch it. Will started to regress in all areas—physically, emotionally, and intellectually. Potty trained more than a year ago, now at four and a half years old, he started having accidents so frequently we were forced to bring the pull-ups back. He'd been proudly drinking out of a big boy cup for months and now could hardly take a sip without making a mess. Imagine how he must've felt as we handed him a sippy cup like the one his two-year-old brother was using.

As upsetting as those physical setbacks were, his intellectual regression was way more disturbing. Will could no longer sing his ABCs, and he was having trouble finding his words. His preschool teachers were incredibly supportive, but he was clearly not doing so well in school anymore. Thankfully, he didn't seem to be having as many seizures at school as he did at home, but he was often tired, disoriented, and irritable. It was tough, but we decided it would be best to pull him out of school. I felt awful taking him from a place he enjoyed going to so much. He loved his teachers, and I knew he would really miss his friends. We had no idea how long we'd need to keep him out, so we tried not to make a big deal about it. His teachers told the other students that Will was sick and promised he would return to class as soon as he was better. The kids decided to make Will a bunch of get-well cards, which was so sweet and thoughtful of them. However, it ended up confusing Will. He looked through the cards and said, "Why did my friends make me these cards for me? I'm not sick." Will would always say he just had bad guys in his brain that he vowed to do battle with. In the end, he was sad to leave his preschool, but we really felt that it was for the best. We needed to focus on getting him well, and we needed to do it immediately.

It turned out to be the right decision. As things continued to get worse, it was best for the both of us that Will was at home. For me, because I felt the need to keep my eyes glued to him at all times, and for Will, because he was in the comfort of his own home. He was unstable on his feet—experiencing up to 50 seizures a day! It was hard to do anything more than stare at him all day and try to keep him safe. Once again, poor little Blake was caught in the middle as the three of us spent every waking minute together in the same room. If I had to use the bathroom, along came Will and Blake. If I wanted to go and get the mail or water the plants outside, along they came. I had to plan my day just right if I wanted to get a shower. I either got up extra early so that Brian could keep an eye on Will, or I waited until he got home from work.

I became awkwardly accustomed to the seemingly endless number of drop and absence seizures Will experienced throughout the course of each day. I hated that he was seizing all day but at the same time I was thankful. He hadn't had another grand mal seizure since our last stay in the hospital, and I prayed he wouldn't have another. Not only are they frightening to witness, but they can also be very dangerous. I had learned through my research that if Will were to have one in his sleep lasting longer than five minutes, he could suffer irreversible brain damage as a result. Thank goodness I kept the boys' video baby monitor as it became a lifeline for me each night.

Most nights I'd spend 15 minutes just staring at the little screen, searching for the faintest sign of a pending grand mal seizure. Often, I'd break down and just climb into Will's bed. The closeness of being curled up beside him gave me the peace of mind I needed, and I was able to get at least a little rest despite the way Will tossed and turned in his sleep as his body and brain tried to rest. The constant vigilance and lack of sleep were really beginning to take a toll.

Then one morning around 4 a.m., one of my worst fears came to life. I heard that unmistakable sound, the same one I'd heard a month before at Children's Hospital, coming out of Will. It was the distinctive sound of a grand mal seizure. It's so hard to explain it in words, but it's guttural, and terrifying, and something I never want to hear again.

As soon as I heard it, I woke Brian up, and we flew to Will's room in an instant. We found him there convulsing in the middle of his bed. It was the kind of seizure that most people think of when they hear the word *epilepsy*. His eyes were rolled back in his head, he had drool dripping out of his mouth, and his entire body was lost in a fit—jerking and jolting uncontrollably. It was a terrible sight to see, not only because we feared for his well-being but because of the sheer helplessness we felt in that moment. He was having a grand mal seizure, and there was nothing we could do to stop it. But now, we knew what we could do to help. Brian looked at the clock and started to count the time as I grabbed the Diastat that we kept close at hand for just this type of emergency, ready to administer it if the seizure lasted past the five-minute mark. Shortly after two minutes had elapsed, Will stopped seizing. Thank God! I just wanted to hug him and tell him it would be alright, but then the tears started to fall, and I couldn't control myself. Not wanting to upset him more, I stepped out of the room to gather myself while Brian—with his calming demeanor and unquestionable strength—spoke quietly to Will, gently coaxing him out of his state of confusion. It was a devastating turn of events. We subjected our son to all this medicine in the hopes that one of them would calm his brain and make the seizures stop. Instead, they increased in number and worsened in intensity all while our son continued to slide backwards, reverting to a toddler's level of development instead of getting ready to enter kindergarten with his peers.

The very next day we were supposed to go on our annual Halloween hayride with a bunch of our high school friends and their children. It's an event we always enjoyed and looked forward to each year. Not this time. Still frazzled from the night before, I called my girlfriend and explained that we were too nervous to bring Will along because his seizures seemed to be getting much worse. The boys were sad to miss this great outing, but I promised we'd go again one day.

It saddened me that we had to miss so many social outings and parties, but our lives had changed dramatically in a short period of time. We still had a lot to figure out. It's moments like that, when we could no longer do things we once so freely did, that made us realize just how much we took for granted. It's natural of course, the whole *you don't know what you've got until it's gone* mentality. Except it wasn't just reserved for missing out on events and trips for us anymore. Eating dinner at the table as a family was no longer an option. Will's drop seizures had gotten so bad that, for him, sitting at a table had become downright dangerous. The threat of continuously hitting his head was no longer worth trying to maintain the routine and stability of sitting together to share a meal. Will was covered in bruises and cuts, so we decided to have picnic dinners together instead. Will ate every meal on the floor, and thought it was pretty cool at first. We got him his own picnic blanket and a special tray that stood on legs for him to use. When he wasn't up for a picnic, we'd let him eat using a tray in front of the television—something we had previously vowed we'd never let our kids do—but it was safe for him and offered a little bit of a treat to a hapless boy dealing with so much more than he ever deserved. So, we made an exception for our exceptional son.

Dinner time wasn't the only example of how our lives had changed. Every part of our daily lives seemed suddenly rife with obstacles. Will would often have seizures near or on the stairs, so we had to make a new rule that he go down the stairs on his bottom. Riding bikes, swimming, and playgrounds were all out: too dangerous. It was so hard to tell him *no* all the time. He just wanted to have fun and be a kid, but we just couldn't allow it. I felt like I'd become an obsessive, crazy person watching Will like a hawk while our sweet Blake felt largely ignored. It broke my heart to hold them both back: one out of necessity and the other out of circumstance. But during the day, with Brian at work, there was only one of me and only so much I could do.

Thankfully, our parents were a huge help. They would come over and sit with Will and play with Blake so that I could do those simple things I had once taken for granted, like taking a shower or putting away laundry. Brian was also great about giving me a break when he was home from work. An hour at the gym or a quick trip to the store would allow me to escape for a bit. My intuitive girlfriends could always tell when a girls' night out was needed, and it always worked to boost my spirits. Just to be able to see their smiling faces and have a drink together was truly invaluable therapy. We would get through this together, even if it took a village.

But before we could really conquer *it*, we needed to know more specifically what *it* was. At this point, we hadn't been given a formal diagnosis. We'd been told Will had epilepsy, but nothing else. When we pressed the doctor, he hesitated before he finally mentioned the terms Doose syndrome and Lennox-Gastaut syndrome. We didn't have any idea what either of those syndromes were or what that meant for Will, but we were determined to find out. Though it's common knowledge that the worst thing a person can do when diagnosed with an illness is to go to Google for information, we simply couldn't help ourselves. We were desperate for information, and it was lurking right there at our fingertips. In hindsight, I wish I would've heeded the warnings. It was a mistake to go down the Google rabbit hole in search of answers, but the damage had been done and our fears for Will's future continued to grow.

# CHAPTER 6
# THE MEDICATION ROLLER COASTER

When most people think about roller coasters, they envision a thrill ride, climbing steep hills only to race down the other side at top speed. They're supposed to be fun, right? The figurative one that Will was on with his myriad of meds was not, I can assure you of that. Will had already been on Keppra and weaned off, and he'd started both Topamax and Klonopin but they had no positive effect. His seizures were more frequent, more varied, and lasting longer. Obviously, something was seriously wrong—Will's brain was pissed, and so were we. Our little four-year-old had been through the ringer for the last two months and that had to stop. We called the neurologists to let them know just how terrible he was doing. Understanding the gravity of his situation, they told us they needed to see him as soon as possible and would call us back once they had a bed available. When that call came just a few short hours later, they informed us that they needed to admit Will to the hospital for a couple days of continuous observation. Doing so would allow them to study what was happening inside of his brain and determine a better course of treatment since the one we'd been following was obviously not working. I was to pack up and head to Children's Hospital as soon as possible.

As much as I didn't want to pack those bags or hear the sound of our suitcase wheels rumbling through the all-too-familiar hospital hallways, I also couldn't wait to get there. I wanted to get Will the help he so badly needed to feel better and just be a kid again. So, I took a deep breath and started to gather our things. Having spent two nights at Children's for the same kind of observation just one month before, this time I knew what to pack. I pulled the grandpa pj's out of Will's drawer again. You remember— the ones that he had been so excited about before his last hospital sleepover? What they lacked in fashion they made up for in functionality: the buttons allowing the nurses access to the leads on his chest. Next, I filled our bag with special stuffed animals and downy soft blankets, crafts, books, video games, Star Wars figures, and DVDs ... anything and everything I thought might make him feel more comfortable in the relative

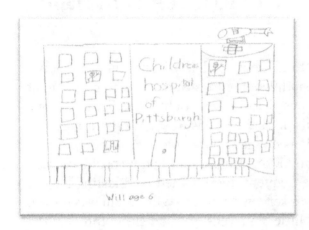

discomfort of his hospital bed. In addition, I'd started to keep a small supply of little prizes in our house that I used to reward the boys or make a bad day a little bit better. So, I packed a couple of new prizes from the stash, figuring they would be appreciated after enduring a blood draw or an IV insertion—all worthy of a prize in my eyes.

As I threw my own things in our overnight bag, I called the grandparents to make arrangements for Blake. Unfortunately, Brian's job as an orthopedic trauma rep isn't flexible. He brings the necessary equipment and assists the surgeon in using it. He works a ton of long hours and is on call on weekends, so he can't easily call off (even when he's sick). He must schedule time off months in advance, so I knew it wasn't even an option to leave Blake home with his daddy. Thank God both sets of parents live close by and are always there when we need them the most. Brian's parents came over in a flash to pick Blake up so that Will and I could head to the hospital ... love them! It was hard to leave our little one behind, but Blake was excited to spend time with his grandparents, and I was relieved he was in good hands.

Making matters even more stressful than they already were, it just so happened that as Will and I made our way to Children's, my parents were also headed to the hospital. My dad was going under the knife for a previously scheduled hip replacement surgery: when it rains it pours. My mom needed to be there for my dad. And while I knew she wanted to take care of her husband; I knew how badly she wanted to be there for her grandsons too. It killed her to not be able to visit Will in the hospital or to help keep an eye on Blake. We promised to keep each other up-to-date from our supportive sentinel posts.

It wasn't long before Will and I arrived at the hospital. A palpable sense of fear and dread washed over me as we made our way through the colorful lobby. Despite the hospital's cheerful décor, I was completely overwhelmed by sadness in that moment. I was sad about what Will would have to endure in the coming days, sad about being surrounded by other afflicted children and their families struggling to survive, sad to be away from

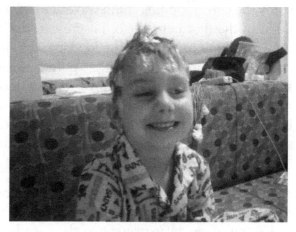

Will still smiling through another EEG!

Blake and Brian, and scared to death that the results of the pending tests would change all our lives in ways I didn't want to even think about. Then, with tears brimming in my eyes, I looked down at Will and saw him smiling from ear to ear.

He asked me excitedly, "Do you think they still have that movie that we watched last time we were here?" A four-year-old's perspective is priceless: so innocent and optimistic. He had no idea what was about to happen, and in a way, I wish I hadn't either.

After we were admitted to the video EEG suite, Will was hooked up to the electrodes once again. We got cozy in our room—our home away from home for the next five days. I unpacked some of Will's things and ordered him some food. After he ate and we started to settle in for the night, the monitors were switched on and I soon enough knew he was in trouble. To help the nurses identify when Will was having a seizure on the video feed, they asked me to press a button every time I saw a change in Will's expression, behavior, or body language. Signs I had grown painfully accustomed to over the last several weeks and could readily recognize. When I pressed the button, the observation team would study the corresponding brain waves recorded by the EEG. At some point in the first hour or so, I'd pressed the button so many times they called out to me over the loudspeaker and said, "Mom, we got it. You don't need to press that button anymore." Will's absence seizures came with blank stares and fluttering eyelids while his multiple myoclonic seizures appeared with a slight head drop or light vocalization. Then there were the generalized grand mal seizures that came with louder vocalization and full body convulsions.

The sheer number of seizures (let alone the varied intensity and duration of each one) revealed during the EEG left little doubt that Will's brain was in worse shape than we had ever imagined. The doctors didn't mince their words when they informed me that extreme measures needed to be taken. Will was immediately treated with more drugs. Ativan via IV was the first drug they administered to try and slow his seizure activity.

After two doses, the seizures continued to come, as did a marked change in Will's behavior. He was agitated and uncomfortable; it was beyond awful to watch. His seizures were coming on so quickly, he was unable to do anything else. The books and crafts we'd brought? I began to wonder if he'd ever be able to play with them again. Poor, sweet Will was like the Andrea Gail in *The Perfect Storm*—a lone ship caught out in a violent sea fighting like hell to just stay afloat in a flurry of monstrous waves. I felt like a seasick passenger on the side of the boat. I felt like I needed to vomit. I didn't know whether it was morning or evening, what day it was, or what time it was ... everything had blurred together, and I hated every minute of it. I felt helpless and hopeless and did the only thing I could as his mother; I laid in his hospital bed and held him close. I cradled my four-and-a-half-year-old son like an infant in my arms and clung to him like my own life depended on it. I felt like we were losing our son, and I wasn't about to let go of him.

I was beyond thankful when Brian was able to get away from work and join us at Children's. We both needed him, and I was flooded with relief when he walked in the door. I couldn't watch Will suffer anymore. Brian wisely sent me on a walk to get some fresh air and clear my head. When I returned, the doctors approached us about trying yet another drug. This time it was IV Depacon. Everything was happening so fast I couldn't even comprehend what they were saying, let alone feel comfortable enough to make any critical decisions. Still, we figured one of the drugs they had was going to work. I mean we were in one of the top children's hospitals in the country and had teams of doctors and nurses working together to try and help our son. They would be able to fix him, right?

As it turned out, the Ativan didn't work, and neither did the Depacon. The next drug they tried was IV Fosphenytoin. We were scared to death. Will was completely incoherent; his body was flooded with a futile cocktail of drugs. We were beside ourselves and had no plan. When the Fosphenytoin also failed, the doctor came in and explained that they had tried everything. There was nothing left to try. *What?* Will lay in his hospital bed, completely out of it, continually seizing, and drooling uncontrollably ... and there was nothing left to do? I was beginning to think I might be in need of a hospital bed myself. I'd lost the ability to function at that point. Thank God Brian was there for us—ever strong—because I didn't have anything left and little Will was beyond fried.

While Will continued to deteriorate, Brian and I once again turned to the internet, researching nonstop and making phone calls whenever we could. We needed as much information as we could get our hands on. We were more desperate than ever to figure this out. We needed to save our son. After what we had witnessed over the past three days, it was clear that Will wasn't responding to available medications. The time had come to explore other avenues of treatment. His neurologist suggested that we move on to dietary treatments to decrease Will's substantial seizure activity. At first glance, the diet appeared to be similar to the Atkins® Diet, which means little to no carbohydrates and lots of fat and protein. I thought, *a diet?* We can do this! Let's get him off these drugs.

Things were finally looking up. We had a new path to pursue, and with it came a new hope. I could hardly wait to get Will out of the hospital and take him back home, but he was so weak and still heavily medicated. So, we stayed put and waited while the drugs began to work their way out of his system. It was during that time that an adorable therapy dog trotted into our room. Will perked up as much as he could when he spotted the dog. The handler asked if it would be OK for the precious lab to visit Will, and I eagerly answered "Yes." Once the dog had sniffed around the room for a moment, she jumped right up on Will's hospital bed and cuddled in by his side. As Will began to pet the dog, I saw him smile and tears streamed down my face (yes, again!). I was done for. After four torturous days, covered with electrodes and hooked up to an IV for hours on end, Will was smiling. *He was smiling!*

Although our stay in the hospital that week had been one of the most horrific experiences of my life, the dedicated staff did their best to make us as comfortable as possible. Once Will was coherent, a life specialist stopped by with a game cart. She was so kind and upbeat. Those volunteers have no idea just how much their service means to the captive hospital patients and their families, all of whom wish they could be anywhere else. Just when we thought that the game cart was the best thing ever, another volunteer arrived with a prize cart! Will couldn't believe that he was allowed to pick anything he wanted from it for *free*. We were getting spoiled and enjoying it.

The following day we were discharged. The electrodes that had been glued to Will's scalp for the past four days were finally removed. He'd been itchy and uncomfortable and was thrilled to have them off. Too bad the glue didn't come off so easily. Even though this wasn't our first rodeo, it was just as frustrating trying to get the matted glue out of Will's hair the second time around. As I helped him get in the shower, I started to seriously think it might be time for a buzz cut. Just as I was about to give up trying to get the sticky stuff out, a sweet nurse stopped in and said that, in her experience, conditioner alone worked best. She was right! I was so happy and thankful to receive her advice, and Will's hair came out better than ever. Yay for small victories!

Though the situation with Will's hair was frustrating, it wasn't as concerning as the fact that my poor boy couldn't stand up on his own two feet. The massive amounts of drugs that he'd been given over the last four days had a major effect on his gross and fine motor skills. To get Will and all our stuff out of the hospital, I needed a wheelchair for my little man. So, with a heavy heart, I strapped him into the wheelchair, grabbed our bags, and headed home. I wished we were leaving with more answers. After all the medications failed to work, Will's neurologist narrowed his diagnosis down to Doose syndrome or Lennox-Gastaut syndrome.

Wanting to know more, we searched the web and found important information on the Doose Syndrome Epilepsy Alliance website.

Myoclonic-atonic Epilepsy (MAE), or Doose syndrome, is an epilepsy syndrome of early childhood that is often resistant to medication (efractory). For this reason, it can be difficult to treat. Doose syndrome is idiopathic generalized epilepsy, meaning that there is no known cause for the seizures (idiopathic) and the seizures originate from all over the brain (generalized) as opposed to coming from one focal area. The onset of Doose syndrome occurs commonly in the first five years of life, with the mean age being three. Statistics show that it usually affects children who have previously developed normally, and boys are twice as likely as girls to develop Doose syndrome.[2]

Here is what we found about Lennox-Gastaut syndrome on the Johns Hopkins All Children's Hospital website.

Lennox-Gastaut syndrome (LGS) is a seizure disorder. Children with LGS will have:

- several different kinds of seizures
- some degree of intellectual disability
- abnormal findings on an EEG (a test to see brain waves/electrical activity)

LGS begins in children when they're 3 to 5 years old. It's a lifelong condition that requires a high level of care.[3]

With this limited knowledge in hand, and no certainty as to which disorder we might actually be dealing with, all we could do

---

[2] "Myoclonic-atonic Epilepsy (MAE)," https://doosesyndrome.org/newly-diagnosed/basic-information/

[3] "Lennox-Gastaut Syndrome," https://www.hopkinsallchildrens.org/patients-families/health-library/healthdocnew/lennox-gastaut-syndrome

was hope and pray for the best. We wanted to get our precious Will back and were determined to do so no matter his diagnosis. We would not give up! We had a chance to try and regulate his seizures through a specified diet and I was already making a mental shopping list of all the things we'd need from the store on the drive home from the hospital. For the first time in a long time, I didn't feel so helpless. I could purchase and prepare the foods that could help Will feel better. I felt positive and hopeful, ready to roll up my sleeves and get to work.

# Chapter 7
## Sayonara Sugar

Coming home after our harrowing five-day hospital stay felt so soothing and safe, our harbor in the tempest. Thankfully, Blake had been in great hands at Grandma and G-Daddy's house while we were on the extended hospital sleepover. Will and I were thrilled to be reunited with Brian and Blake and even more elated to be away from all the doctors, nurses, needles, and drugs. To add to our abundant joy, my parents had also just come home from their stay in the hospital, my dad the proud owner of a brand a new hip. They were anxious to see the boys, so they hobbled over to visit as soon as possible. My mom felt terrible that she had her own patient to tend to and couldn't stick around to make everything better like she usually would, her superhero grandparent role on temporary hiatus.

My parents were saddened to see the state Will was in. He was in a fog, and his ability to walk and talk was still distinctly compromised. The heavy mixture of medications he'd been given in the hospital continued to course through his body, and we knew he wouldn't be able to function properly until they wore off completely. I could tell my parents were upset as they tried their best to conceal the fear that was undoubtedly brewing inside. Their sweet, innocent, four-year-old grandson was seriously sick with an illness we still couldn't definitively name and that had defied all traditional treatments. No wonder they were freaking out—we all were. Luckily, my sister and her three kids showed up soon after my parents did and managed to lighten the mood. The boys always enjoy spending time with their cousins!

Next to arrive was Will's best friend, Jack. Will was still unstable, so he was sitting on the floor in the family room when Jack arrived. Jack must've realized that Will couldn't get up as he immediately plopped down right next to him on the floor. After asking Will a couple of questions, to which he didn't respond, Jack quickly gleaned that Will wasn't able to say much either. Instead of backing away from an awkward and uncomfortable situation like so many adults are prone to do,

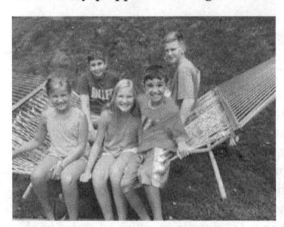

Front row left to right: Lily, Mia, Blake

Back row left to right: Will, Luke

that witty four-year-old decided to start cracking jokes! Jack turned to Will with a goofy grin and blurted, "Hey Will, do you want to see my underpants?" Will might not have been able to answer with words, but his resounding giggles and a genuine smile were answer enough. Jack and Will must've spent the next hour belly laughing together on the floor. Their laughter was infectious, and Jack's mom and I got caught up in the hysteria chuckling right along with them. In moments like that, I had to acknowledge that there is definitely some truth to the adage, *laughter is the best medicine*. Jack's visit was the absolute best therapy around and we were thrilled to have him for as long as he wanted to stay.

Despite all of the stress and chaos surrounding Will's condition, the world continued to spin, and life went on. It just so happened that two short days after we'd returned home from the hospital, was Blake's second birthday. It was a happy occasion to celebrate with family and an opportunity to give our little guy some of the attention he'd been so sorely missing as a bystander to his big brother's trauma. Thankfully, Blake had always been a happy-go-lucky child who handled adversity well. After opening an early birthday present and playing with his cousins for a spell, Blake had forgotten any *slight* he might've felt in the prior week and had acted as though nothing out of the ordinary had ever happened.

Will sure did miss his friends. It had been a month since we'd pulled him out of school with no real hope of him being able to return anytime soon. There were still traces of the medication lingering in his blood and he was still having a lot of seizures. On top of that, he'd just started on the Atkins Diet, and I had to prepare all his completely carbohydrate-free meals and snacks and watch him eat every bite. The prospect of leaving the house together was terrifying, let alone the thought of leaving him off for even a few hours at his preschool.

Thankfully, Will seemed to be tolerating the new diet and with the help of the internet and a couple of books, so following it wasn't all that difficult. It was a little tough on me since I don't eat meat, but my preferences and quirks don't mean a thing when it comes to my son's health. It took me no more than a passing thought before I got used to making meals for Will that consisted almost entirely of meat. His plates weren't particularly colorful (think brown beef and bland chicken breasts), so I tried to make it more appetizing and fun by cutting the food into interesting shapes and sizes and arranging them into Will's own little dietary dioramas.

Will had been out of the hospital for one week before Halloween was upon us. It figures, a holiday celebrated with ungodly amounts of candy and junk food falls seven days after my four-year-old gets put on a low/no sugar diet. It was time to get creative! So, after some thought and googling, we decided to allow Will to go trick-or-treating with his friends and to exchange all the candy he collected for inedible prizes instead. Once the costumes were on and Will and Blake were ready to go, we realized that Will was still too physically weak to go door to door. Thanks to some quick thinking on Brian's part, we grabbed our wagon out of the shed and acted like it was the plan all along. I said, "Boys, hop in! We're going to take you for a fun ride around the neighborhood."

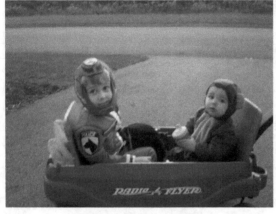

Halloween wagon time!

Will got out of the wagon here and there and made the trek to ring a few doorbells.

The one house I went to with him, the owner said, "Go ahead and grab two pieces."

Will replied, "No thanks, I am on a diet!"

The guy burst out laughing, and so did I. Will couldn't understand what was so funny about what he'd, said but he just shrugged and went back to the wagon.

One of the best parts of Halloween is returning home and dumping the abundant haul onto the floor, taking an inventory of all the goodies, trading favorites, and allowing the parents to pilfer a piece or two. Not that year. As soon as we returned home, I quickly set up a Halloween store, laying out an assortment of small prizes and one large LEGO set for Will to choose from. He decided to trade his candy stash in for the LEGO set he'd had on his wish list. Turns out that all the anxiety and guilt we felt about Will missing out on the traditional Halloween treats was all for not. He did awesome. He got to dress up, said "Trick-or-Treat," and was thrilled to get a LEGO set! Blake was equally excited about the mountain of candy that he had collected, and Brian and I were ecstatic that both of our boys had a good holiday and were genuinely happy. We learned to appreciate those moments in the sun—those fleeting times when all felt right in the world. When you don't know what's ahead from one day, one hour, one minute to the next, you have to try and live in the moment.

Our collective family happiness ebbed and flowed over the next couple months. Will had good days and bad days. But as the weeks went by, we were relieved to see that the Atkins Diet seemed to be helping. Instead of 30 seizures a day, he averaged 15. Still far too many in my eyes, so we battled on.

Given the experimental nature of the dietary approach, we worked closely with the neurology team at Children's Hospital to measure ongoing progress and determine next steps. We met monthly with a dedicated neurologist and dietician to review Will's seizure log and daily diet diary to track trends and make adjustments. He got bloodwork often to monitor his medication levels as well as his key nutrient concentrations. To aid in the process, we were given our own personal blood monitoring kit similar to what someone with diabetes would use. I used the kit to prick his finger once a month or as needed to check his blood ketone level. We were also to use ketone sticks to test Will's urine daily. If you've ever tried the Atkins Diet, then you know all about ketones. For anyone who hasn't, ketones are produced when your body is using fat for energy instead of glucose. That is the main goal of the Atkins Diet, and we were told those same ketones had the potential to calm Will's brain and decrease his seizure activity.

Because the Atkins Diet isn't as nutritionally well rounded as a growing child's diet should be, Will also needed to take a host of supplements to give him the nutrients his limited food supply could not. He needed extra calcium, magnesium, and a sugar-free multivitamin. Thankfully, we had the best pharmacy in the world, and they were a god send to us. They were there for us from the beginning and have always gone above and beyond to help us find what we needed, when we needed it. I never imagined just how hard it would be to find sugar-free children's medicines and vitamins until we needed them. Sugar is in absolutely everything!

Beyond the obvious—candy, cakes, and fruit-flavored drinks—we discovered there is sugar lurking everywhere. Toothpaste, shampoo, lotion, sunscreen, hand sanitizer ... you name it, it probably has sugar in it. Some days I felt like a C.S.I. (concealed sugar investigator) on the hunt for products that were 100% sugar-free. We were determined to get Will's daily seizure number down to zero and if that meant scouring every health food store and internet retailer to do it, then that's what we'd do. *Sayonara sugar!*

# CHAPTER 8
# NO CHUCK E. CHEESE FOR US

Thanksgiving and Christmas came and went with relative quiet. Things began to settle down as Will adjusted to his new dietary restrictions. It was quite the challenge during a holiday season celebrated with an abundance of decadent dishes and traditional treats. Thankfully, it's also a time of year when the centerpiece of each meal is protein: turkey, ham, and beef galore. We were committed to sticking with the plan and hopeful it would help. By the time the New Year rolled around, we felt that Will was stable enough to head back to preschool after taking the fall semester off. January is the time for new beginnings, right?

On his first morning back to school, Will ran into our bedroom at 5:30 a.m. fully dressed, including shoes. He was so excited to go back to preschool. Once again, I would've been hesitant if it weren't for the incredible group of teachers I was trusting for Will's care. It bears repeating how safe I felt knowing that Will's teacher was a retired nurse and 100% capable of administering his rectal emergency seizure medication if needed. His teachers and classmates welcomed Will back with open arms and heartfelt enthusiasm. He felt so special and the wide smile on his face confirmed in my mind that we were doing the right thing in sending him back.

But while Will nearly bounced into the building each day, I was a nervous wreck. Some days I felt so anxious that I'd spend the entire two and a half hours he was in class sitting in my car in the parking lot. I thought it'd be for the best if I stayed close by ... just in case. Then there were other days when I'd get a little adventurous, spending only half the time in the parking lot. When I felt particularly daring, I would drop him off and head to a nearby trail and take a walk. Then one day in March I decided it'd be OK if I ran to the mall to pick up a birthday gift. I'd just arrived at the store when I received a frantic call from the preschool director. "Will has fallen and hit his head," she said. "We think you should come and get him as soon as possible."

This had been my fear for the last two months; it was the reason I'd camped out in the parking lot all those weeks. Of course, the moment I gave in to the false sense of security that those incident-free weeks gave me, Will got hurt, and I was a good ten-minute drive away. I rushed back to get him, silently cursing at myself the entire way for being so foolish and for getting too comfortable. When I arrived back at school, I was flooded with relief when he looked to be OK. His teachers thought he might've had a drop seizure while sitting at the art table that caused him to hit his head. In the grand scheme of things, it was just a little scrape—nothing that our family hadn't unfortunately grown accustomed to of late— but it still shook me to the core. I knew then that I couldn't relax, couldn't take a string of good days for granted and assume calm seas and smooth sailing ahead. To this day, and probably for the rest of our lives to be honest, I've got my guard up just waiting for the next storm to strike while praying that it never comes. It might seem sad or even fatalistic, but when you're dealing with something as unpredictable as Will's condition, I knew I needed to expect the worst and hope for the best.

In the days that followed, Will's seizures seemed to be less frequent and less severe. At the same time though, he'd been falling far too frequently for my liking. The week after he hit his head at school, a big snowstorm hit, and we were playing around in our family room enjoying the view of our backyard blanketed in white. Without warning, Will fell and this time we weren't sure if it was due to a seizure or just to being a kid! Either way, he hit the corner of his eye pretty hard, and it wouldn't stop bleeding. The roads were completely covered with snow and the forecast called for a couple more inches to come. So, rather than braving the bad roads and heading downtown to Children's Hospital, we decided to go to the local ER. We threw on our winter coats and I climbed into the backseat between the boys' car seats before we set off, and Brian carefully maneuvered our car over the hilly, unplowed streets of our neighborhood. It was slow going but we arrived at the ER safely.

Luckily the cut wasn't very deep, so the ER doctor was able to just glue the skin back together. Will was such a trooper; he never even flinched while the nurse fixed him up. He shrugged and told her he'd been through much worse. Well, he wasn't wrong about that. Not long after he was all patched up, we were discharged from the ER. Will seemed to be utterly amazed that we didn't have to have a sleepover, and we were all thrilled to be headed home. As we approached the house, we were pleasantly surprised to find three of our wonderful neighbors shoveling the driveway for us! I'll say it a million times over, we have been blessed with the best neighbors in the world. Will also found a care package on the front porch filled with prizes to cheer him up. It was such a nice surprise for all of us, especially Will. So much so, that he immediately forgot about the trip to the ER and moved on to pour over his new loot!

And thus, we managed to make it through the long, cold winter without any other drama. It was refreshing to have so many mundane days pass by. Though I was always a little anxious, I was ecstatic that we hadn't needed to make any trips to the hospital and relieved to be free of any kind of highly emotional situations. Spring was finally here as was Will's highly anticipated fifth birthday.

Will decided he wanted to have a pirate-themed party at our house. Thank goodness he didn't ask to have a party at Chuck E. Cheese like most five-year-olds. Not only was pizza off the menu for Will, but so was sitting at a table to eat. The events that unfolded under our own roof the day of the party would have been a total nightmare in the raucous, overcrowded rooms of hyperactive kids at Chuck E. Cheese.

The day of Will's party was an unusually hot afternoon in May. Heat was not Will's friend. He'd always had a hard time with it, but it seemed that the meds he was taking made matters worse. Knowing that, we always tried to avoid hot, stressful environments. But with 15 excited kids slated to attend Will's pirate party, I knew that would be nearly impossible. Will did very well at first, playing and laughing with the other kids, but it wasn't long before the sweltering heat and the natural noise levels that occur at kids'

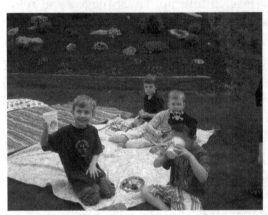

Will's fifth birthday party (pirate picnic)

parties got to Will, and his brain decided to shut down. Will went limp during a drop seizure at the kitchen island and promptly banged his head off the edge of the hard countertop. A couple of his guests and their moms witnessed the whole thing and were stunned silent with shock. Of course, his seizures were nothing new to me but having them happen in front of a crowd of concerned and caring onlookers was. I felt sad for Will as I picked him up off the stool and carried him to the couch. His friends all gathered around while he recovered from his seizure. They were clearly worried, but not put off, and ready to welcome Will back to his own party. Meanwhile, my mom, sister, and amazing friends started to clean up the mess that we'd made. I helped Will open his gifts as I held a cold compress to his forehead. I couldn't help but think in that moment, *thank God we're not at Chuck E. Cheese*!

With Will's birthday behind us, the long days of summer were quickly approaching. I knew it'd be a challenging season, especially with his increased propensity for suffering from heat stroke. Still, we kept on living and planned on a few fun trips and activities, ever mindful of Will's issues and limitations. So, when our neighbors and good friends invited us to go to Niagara Falls for the weekend, we gladly accepted. We all needed a little fun in our lives! It was an effort to get all of Will's meds, supplements, and Atkins Diet food packed up for the trip but the excitement the kids had over going away certainly outweighed all the hassle.

The drive to the falls was uneventful and our time spent there with our neighbors was wonderful. From the Maid of the Mist boat tour to the gigantic indoor waterpark, the kids had a total blast! The parents managed to have some grown-up fun as well. Our friends are big wine connoisseurs, and they brought a bunch of wine with them to sample. We found a lovely little gazebo right outside of our hotel rooms that we quickly commandeered. The baby monitor I brought along was even able to work from the gazebo, so we could laugh and chat and just relax with our friends. It was just what we needed to unwind and recharge!

By the last day of our stay, Will was exhausted. I knew we'd probably pushed his limits, but Brian and I were banking on him sleeping the whole way home. There was still a little more fun that we could fit in, and we decided to go for it. We hit an arcade, played a round of mini golf, and then grabbed lunch. When we sat down to eat, Will's cheeks were bright red, and I could tell he was going downhill. Brian went back to the hotel to fetch the car, so I decided to take the boys across the street to get one last look at the falls while we waited for Brian to pick us up. The second we stepped foot on the small and crowded overlook, Will started to vomit everywhere. I had Blake in my arms and no purse, no napkins, nothing at all to help clean him up. It was upsetting and a little embarrassing, not because Will was throwing up everywhere, but because I was so ill prepared for the whole thing.

I just stood there helpless and watched him wretch while clutching Blake to my chest. I was so grateful when a sweet mother who had little ones of her own tossed me a container of wipes without getting too close. I thanked her profusely and did my best to clean up what I could with two crying boys in my arms. When Brian pulled up five minutes later to find us all crying, he couldn't imagine what had happened. We rushed into the car and held our breaths hoping he wouldn't be sick the whole way back to Pittsburgh.

After the horrific scene at the falls, we decided to inquire about changing his medications. Will was tired of *losing his arms and legs* (fainting) and the nausea that accompanied his far too frequent heat strokes. We were less than enthused when his doctors suggested using a different drug that was newer to the market. I hated what all the drugs he'd tried to this point had done to him and I wasn't up for another trial: too many unknown side effects with no assurance that it would actually help with his seizures. But, after a lot of research and thorough discussions, Brian and I decided to give it a go. We were hopeful that it could help him and that feeling was enough to move forward with his doctor's plan.

Sadly, it didn't take long for us to discover that the new drug wasn't the answer we were looking for. In fact, it actually made Will feel worse—as usual. He started experiencing more seizures and more heatstroke episodes; he had trouble sleeping and started having bloody noses. He could no longer spend any time outside because it exhausted him completely. That meant no more baseball, no more going to the park, no more than 20 minutes outside ... period. It was ridiculous and disheartening, and we knew that it couldn't go on. We weaned Will off the new medication and decided to look for other alternatives. There had to be a better way, and we were determined to do whatever it took to find out what that was.

# CHAPTER 9
# A SECOND OPINION

*"Fear can hold you prisoner. Hope can set you free."*[4]

*- Stephen King*

When in doubt or even disbelief, it's wise to get a second opinion. Several months and too many seizures to count, and Will's diagnosis was still as nebulous and mystifying as the human brain itself. How were we supposed to feel confident that we were doing everything in our power to help our son when we had so many unanswered questions regarding his condition? Our doctor was aware that we were seeking another opinion and supported our quest. Brian and I got to work researching specialists until we found the doctor we wanted to see. He was a leader in pediatric epilepsy treatments and had been well published in the medical journals. With his impressive list of credentials, I figured it would be impossible to get an appointment. When we were finally ready to reach out to this doctor, my fears were confirmed. The wait list to secure an appointment was extremely and dishearteningly long.

I was desperate and despondent and the nurse who'd answered the call must have heard it in my voice. We'd already tried every conventional course of treatment available and none of them had worked. Our son was regressing, and we had hit a wall. We were trying like hell not to feel hopeless and refusing to believe that we'd run out of options. Just then, the nurse threw me a lifeline.

---

[4] Stephen King, "Different Seasons,"
https://www.goodreads.com/quotes/441313-fear-can-hold-you-prisoner-hope-can-set-you-free

She said, "Mrs. Simmons, how about I give you the doctor's email and you can present your case that way? He's extremely helpful to patients and families all over the world, communicating via email."

I fully admit I was skeptical. I thought there was no way that this extremely busy, sought-after physician would respond to an email from me, a complete stranger seeking counsel without compensation. Will wasn't his patient. What were the odds he'd even read it, let alone reply? At the same time, I thought, *What have I got to lose?*

After getting the boys to sleep that night, I sat down with my computer and drafted a lengthy message. Then I redrafted it not once, but twice. Details were important and each time I got close to pressing the send button, I'd remember something else I thought might be critical for his consideration. Finally, I told myself, *Enough!* I wanted to be thorough, not annoying, and I felt like I was getting dangerously close to the latter.

At 10 p.m., I closed my eyes and hit send. A surge of energy rushed through my body like a shot of adrenaline. As I stared at my *Sent* mailbox, with a hitch in my breath, I realized what it was that had me feeling so unnerved—it was *hope*. It'd been so long since we'd genuinely had any that I almost didn't recognize it. This one doctor could hold the key to finally unlocking Will's condition, ending his seizures, and relieving our uncertainty. Despite my sudden swell of optimism, I knew the odds of this renowned physician replying to my random email were slim at best. So, you might imagine my complete surprise when just 30 short minutes later I received a response. We were floored to have been given a concrete answer. He said, "In my professional opinion, I would proceed to the ketogenic diet."

Will had been on the Atkins Diet for seizure control for the past nine months. In that time, it had helped reduce the number of seizures he experienced by 50%. It was progress, but naturally, we wanted Will to be 100% seizure free. This doctor believed that the ketogenic diet could get him there.

Being on the ketogenic diet requires even more precision and discipline than following the Atkins plan. Our initial research revealed that starting on a true keto diet typically requires the participant to be admitted to a hospital so the patient can be weaned off food completely for a couple of days in a controlled environment. In essence, by pursuing this path we were consenting to starve our son. It was heartbreaking to even think about putting him through that process. Food had been one of the only safe things Will could rely on since his seizures had started, and now, we were going to intentionally deprive him. The doctors explained to us that removing food would allow Will to be in a state of ketosis quicker. Our bodies begin to burn fat stores when carbohydrates and protein are not available. When that process happens, ketones are created, and the brain is happy to burn those for energy instead. It is believed that the brain is calmer when running on ketones instead of glucose and thus, the number of seizures lessens in that environment. The true mechanisms of the diet are still a mystery but its efficiency in lessening seizure activity has been proven many times.

Brian kept digging and did some extra research as he reviewed those trials and studies. I am so lucky to have such a strong partner in this fight. He reasoned that Will had already been living on a restricted diet for the past nine months with fewer seizures to show for it. He was already producing ketones, we just needed to step it up. The ketogenic diet is about precision and measuring and giving the body and brain exact amounts of fat, protein, and carbohydrates. It was going to require diligence, discipline, and tenacity. But if it could be the difference in helping our son beat this disorder, then nothing would stop us from trying. Once again, due to the experimental nature of this kind of homeopathic treatment, Will would continue to take his anti-seizure medication. Though none of the meds had been particularly effective, they had to be taken as a safeguard. If all went as well as we hoped, the need to continue taking them would wane right along with Will's seizures.

That night, as we decompressed after having made the decision to pursue the keto diet, I peeked at the baby monitor we still used to keep a watchful eye on Will. He looked so peaceful in the blissful serenity of sleep. I smiled at the image, and that feeling of renewed hope felt awesome. It was time for bed, and for the first time in a long time, I felt like we might actually have a restful night's sleep.

# CHAPTER 10
# A BLESSING IN (A HORRIBLE) DISGUISE

It was the Fourth of July weekend, and we were still full of hope. We were committed to trying the keto diet. All that remained was choosing a date to admit Will to the hospital to get him started. Since it was a holiday, we decided to live it up and enjoy ourselves before the dreaded day arrived and all the dietary denial that would follow.

The weather that morning was absolutely perfect. We decided to start the day by taking a leisurely walk on a peaceful, scenic bike trail. Because my parents lived close to the trail, Nonny decided to join us. Following our little stroll, the boys wanted to spend some time exploring the woods and a slow-moving creek near the entrance to the trail. Being in no particular rush, that's exactly what we did. They ran around the edge of the creek, skipped stones across its shimmering surface, and peered into the rippling water in search of well-camouflaged fish. It was a glorious day to be out in nature and the kids were having a blast!

After our morning on the trail, the boys were understandably hungry. Knowing that Will would soon be on a very restricted diet, it didn't take much for them to convince me to stop at McDonalds for a breakfast sandwich and some time on their outdoor playground. In line with the Atkins Diet, I ordered a sausage biscuit for the boys to share: Will got the sausage and Blake got the biscuit. After they ate, they shucked their shoes and headed for the slide, crawling through a maze of colorful tunnels, and running around until they were too hot to keep going. Time for the pool.

My sister and her family belonged to a country club down the street, and they invited us to meet them for a swim. Will and Blake just adore their cousins and all the kids had a wonderful time playing together in the pool. As we headed home from a long day of fun, exhaustion began to set in. The boys were asleep the instant their heads hit their pillows, and Brian and I took advantage of the quiet summer night to enjoy a glass of wine together and catch up on our days. Unfortunately, he'd been at work all day and missed out on our Fourth of July fun.

It was right around midnight when I heard soft noises emanating from the monitor in Will's room. When I took a peek, I was surprised to see how extremely restless Will seemed to be, especially considering how tired he must have been. After a couple minutes, he started to whimper and that's when I decided I'd feel more comfortable by his side for the rest of the night. So, I turned off the monitor, grabbed my pillow and headed into his room. The second I laid down beside him, I could feel the heat radiating off his tiny body. It was obvious that he had a fever. I got up immediately and headed downstairs to grab his Motrin pills. Most five-year-olds take liquid pain reliever; it tastes pretty good and goes down easy. Because of the Atkins Diet, Will didn't have that option, as those formulas are comprised of mostly sugar. I was glad he was able to swallow the pills and did so without complaint.

The Motrin had been in his system for a full 30 minutes, but his fever continued to climb. It was getting close to 104°F, and I was terrified. A fever that high can be dangerous to anyone, but in Will's case it was particularly frightening as that kind of temperature increase often triggered more seizures and more frequently. He really didn't need that kind of collateral damage at that point, but I knew that if we couldn't bring his fever down, that's exactly what he'd get.

We put him in a cool bath and sponged him down to bring down his fever. When that too failed, I decided to ring the neurologist on call. It was now 2 a.m., and Will was still burning up—a listless wet noodle that couldn't be farther from the happy, active boy who'd just spent his day laughing and playing in the warm summer sun. I wasn't surprised when the neurologist told us to get him to Children's as fast as we could. Ever calm and collected, Brian sensed my growing hysteria and decided it'd be best if we took Will downtown together. So, while I got our things together, Brian dialed my parents and arranged for them to take Blake. Thank God we live close to one another and that our families are always willing to help.

When we arrived at the ER, I was pleasantly surprised by the welcome wagon waiting for Will. No sign-in process or a typical three-hour ER wait. I guess it's a fortunate perk of being an unfortunate regular. At that point, I was just relieved that they were ready for Will and able to get him hooked up to an IV right away to prevent dehydration. Shortly after they ran the line, things took a turn for the worse. In addition to the fever that had landed him in the hospital, Will's stomach began to revolt, wracking his body with both violent bouts of diarrhea and uncontrollable vomiting. If all of that weren't bad enough, our sweet, beleaguered boy started to have the seizures we'd feared would follow along with the fever.

It was the worst medical situation I had ever witnessed. As his body continued to roil and revolt, Will was reduced to a weary rag doll, too spent, and afflicted to make it to the bathroom. Much to his chagrin, Will was fitted with a small adult diaper and a basin was placed by his head. As I stood by, horrified and helpless, I couldn't help but wonder how this could be the same boy who—less than 24 hours earlier—had been contentedly splashing in the pool with his brother and cousins. What was happening to our sweet Will, and why was it happening? The doctors were just as baffled as we were. Will's symptoms were all over the place and his fever refused to let up.

With no clear answers in sight and obvious cause for concern, his neurologist decided to order a bunch of blood work and change his medications. They added a drug called Klonopin to his repertoire and removed a recently prescribed drug, Banzel, that he'd only been on for two weeks. Another medication gone out the window. We hadn't noticed any marked improvement during the time he'd been on it anyway. In fact, he'd been experiencing a host of side effects we weren't too pleased about: trouble sleeping, twitching eyes, and impaired balance ... so much for Banzel being a possible miracle drug. Another failure was not what we wanted for Will. He was beyond sick, and we were beyond worried.

On our third day in the hospital, Will finally turned the corner. He stopped vomiting and his fever finally broke. And at 10 a.m., as I lay in the hospital bed beside him, I realized that I hadn't witnessed one seizure since we'd been awake. Could it be true? It felt like someone had flipped a switch turning all of Will's symptoms off as swiftly as they had started. Knowing that he was out of imminent danger, Brian and I began to focus on other aspects of his health. We realized that Will hadn't had one thing to eat for the last four days. Naturally, our thoughts shifted to feeding our son and that's when it hit us ... Will was in starvation mode; thanks to whatever horrific illness he'd just been blessed with. His body put itself in ketosis. Will started the ketogenic diet without even trying to. If every dark cloud has a silver lining, then this was definitely ours—a miracle born from mayhem.

We were all still perplexed about how he'd gotten so sick. Was it just a horrible stomach bug? Then we realized we didn't care; he *wasn't* seizing! He started to perk up a little bit and we were extremely grateful. We had been in freak-out mode for the last four days, and our baby was coming around. His team of doctors and dietician confirmed what we hoped and prayed had happened because of this otherwise awful experience. Will was officially on the ketogenic diet with no need to fast! He'd inadvertently put himself into ketosis and was ready to go. We agreed to keep Will on one medication (Depakote) during the course of his ketogenic diet but would wean him off of all others. We could hardly contain our excitement.

Though Will was on the road to recovery, his stomach was still unsteady, so they kept him in diapers and on the IV while he continued to recuperate. Meanwhile, his designated dietician scheduled a time for me to get some much-needed training in the kitchen. Given the research I'd already done, I knew that facilitating the ketogenic diet wasn't going to be easy. Although I was an exercise science and sports nutrition major at Virginia Tech, and had some knowledge in the area already, I knew I still had much to learn.

I never imagined I'd be taking a cooking class in a hospital kitchen but that's exactly what I was about to do. I was eager to learn and ready to get this show on the road. As I took the employee elevator to the depths of Children's Hospital, I was filled with a renewed sense of hope and excitement. Was this the answer we had been searching for? After multiple drugs failed to help, would this strict diet be Will's saving grace? I closed my eyes and prayed that this would be the winning treatment. Please ketogenic diet do *not* let us down!

The cooking course was very helpful, and the dietician who taught me was amazing. She was not only knowledgeable, but her delivery was kind and endearing. She was one of our favorite people to see whenever we had to visit Children's Hospital. She trained under the group at Johns Hopkins, so she was filled with tons of information and some extremely useful tips. Together, we weighed, measured, and prepared Will's meals for the rest of the day. He was going to be in shock when he realized his new portions sizes are fit for an ant. Breakfast consisted of one egg mixed with one fourth of a cup of cream and one third of a stick of butter. Lunch was going to be a keto shake and three slices of avocado and dinner was 30 grams of steak served with a half a cup of broccoli and one cup of heavy cream frozen. It was shocking to me just how little he was going to be allowed to eat on this diet. The goal of the plan is to remove carbohydrates and most proteins from the diet leaving fat as the major source of energy.

I thought the Atkins Diet was difficult for a five-year-old. Will was going to be eating some unappetizing food for the next 12-24 months. Cream, butter, and oil made up the majority of his meal plan. I continued to pray for him as I quickly realized this was going to be so much more than a diet; this was a new way of life. It was our new reality—one we hoped would help get the *bad guys* out of his brain once and for all.

As I hopped on the elevator after the lesson, I realized I hadn't been outside of the hospital's walls for five full days. It was time to go home. Will's fever was gone, and his intestinal issues were subsiding. With our new game plan in place and his meds straightened out, all I could do was watch and wait for our discharge papers. I missed Brian and Blake dearly and was anxious to get home and get our kitchen prepared for Will's new diet.

When the neurologist came by to dismiss us, I was surprised that they still had no idea what had caused Will to become so sick. I began to wonder if we would ever know. At the end of the day, we realized it didn't matter. I figured it was simply a gift from God. He wanted to show us the way to the best treatment for our sweet, sick Will.

Even though Will felt vastly better he was still too weak to walk. So, I packed everything up and got him situated in a wheelchair for the short journey to our car.

As I wheeled him down the hall, I heard someone screaming, "Mrs. Simmons, wait! Don't leave!" I turned around to see our super sweet resident running down the hall holding a file. She said, "You are never going to believe this!" Will's cultures came back positive for Salmonella poisoning!"

We discussed the ways he might have obtained the poisoning. I mentioned that we had been playing by a creek, swimming in a public pool, and that he had a piece of sausage from McDonalds. I was relieved to know what had made him so sick and to know that his suffering was truly over, so we didn't focus on the source anymore. With me preparing every bite of his food for the foreseeable future, there was no way he'd be getting that again any time soon.

# CHAPTER 11
# WHAT A DIFFERENCE A DIET CAN MAKE

That Fourth of July weekend had been simultaneously the most harrowing and hopeful holiday of my life. We came out on the other side with a new treatment plan in place and a renewed sense of optimism. Fortunately, we still had a lot of summer left which was plenty of time for all of us to adjust to Will's new diet before he started kindergarten. Even though it was still weeks away, I could already feel the tug of amplified anxiety I knew would be present that first day of school. All parents get a little emotional sending their first born out into the world, but I knew I'd be feeling it more than most—not just on that day but likely for the all the days of my life.

Will's condition didn't just change him, it changed me too—as a parent, and as a person. I will never *not* worry about him. I'll always be on high alert, waiting for the next shoe to drop. Not because I'm a defeatist, resigned to a terrible fate, but because years of fear and anxiety had worn a groove in my heart, making me irrevocably paranoid. I've learned to live by the saying, *Prepare for the worst and hope for the best.*

So, I prepared, spending countless hours in my kitchen crafting Will's ketogenic meals. Ten days into his new regimen, and Will was still incredibly seizure-free. We'd been accustomed to him having over ten seizures a day for more than a year, so having one, let alone ten seizure-free days was glorious. I thank God for every seizure-free day, and so does Will. He started to feel more confident as he regained control of his erratic brain. The tangible differences the diet was making weren't lost on Will. He knew that it was helping and loved the way it made him feel. It made the transition much easier than I'd anticipated, and I was thankful I didn't have to force Will to accept it or feel guilty for restricting his diet.

Regardless of how well Will accepted it, ketogenic diets do take a toll on the body. As such, we needed to go to the clinic at

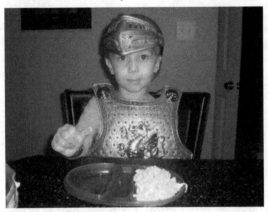

Children's Hospital once a month to monitor his overall health. During these visits, they ran blood tests to check for the development of liver damage, kidney stones, or other troubling symptoms that sometimes accompany a ketogenic diet. While we were thankful his

Our warrior, Will, eating a plate full of cream.

liver and kidneys were functioning fine, it was worrisome (though not unexpected) to learn that Will's cholesterol had gone through the roof. I expected that a diet so high in fat would likely boost his cholesterol levels, but it broke my heart to learn that my five-year-old had a reading of 234.

That was just one of the less-than-desirable side effects Will experienced. He also suffered from constant constipation—a logical outcome of eating a diet so high in fat, so low in fiber, and very few fruits and vegetables. At the dietician's urging, Miralax was added to his list of daily meds and supplements to help relieve that pain. Despite these issues, when we sat down with his neurologist and nurse practitioner (whom we adore!) to review his seizure log, it was worth it all to see the giant goose egg on the page. He hadn't had a single seizure!

Will had become a total champ when getting tests done, particularly blood work. He knew the drill and didn't fight it, never even batting an eye when the needles arrived. He'd just roll up his sleeve and coolly ask, "How many vials today?" like a casual observer might comment on the weather. Always such a trooper; he's simply the best.

There were a couple of tests that Will hadn't yet experienced though that needed to be done at the start of his diet. An electrocardiogram (EKG) and an echocardiogram were ordered to establish a baseline measurement. Will was nervous about taking the tests, but I wasn't too concerned. I assured him that the tests wouldn't be painful or invasive and compared them to the EEG, MRI, and sonograms he'd had in the past.

The test went off without a hitch, but the results were another story. I felt like I'd been hit by a truck when we were told at the appointment that Will's EKG showed a possible problem with his heart. The second after we'd stepped out of the building, I called Brian and burst into tears. I explained between sobbing breaths how the EKG had identified an area of concern.

He was certain that I must've been mistaken saying, "Will had bad EEGs not EKGs. His heart is good, it's his brain we were working on, right?"

I thought it was a bad nightmare, oh how I wish that's all it was. Unfortunately, I knew what I'd heard. It was definitely his heart, and we now needed to see a pediatric cardiologist.

I was thankful that we already knew a great pediatric cardiologist, though the way we'd come to know him was born from tragic circumstances. Our dear friends had lost their son to a heart complication some years ago. They now host an annual memorial golf outing to commemorate their son while raising awareness of the complication that took his life and raising funds for pediatric cardiology research. Brian and I had met this well-known cardiologist at the outing numerous times. I was relieved to know we'd be meeting a familiar face as we forged into unfamiliar territory in a different department at Children's Hospital. The cardiologist was kind and blunt. He said without hesitation that we had nothing to worry about. He told us to put this out of our minds and focus our attentions back on Will's seizure disorder and the diet that had been keeping it at bay. What a relief!

We were ecstatic and ready to celebrate the good news. Time to stop at Dormont Park! Every time we left the hospital, if Will felt up to it, we would stop at the park on our way home. It's a cool, little community park that he associated with feeling good. He coined it *Castle Park* because of the high peaks and wooden structures, and it felt magical that day. As I watched him climb and crawl and laugh and smile, I tried to commit the scene to my memory. His heart was healthy, and we were happy. Thank God!

With Will's heart scare behind us, we spent the next couple of months working on the diet. Now, more than ever, I was so thankful that Brian and I had made the choices and sacrifices needed to enable me to be a stay-at-home mom. Preparing Will's strict ketogenic diet plan was practically a full-time job. I spent hours driving around to different grocery, health food, and specialty stores, gathering a variety of ingredients. He was only allowed to have certain brands, and everything had to be weighed, measured, and eaten in its entirety. He wasn't permitted to miss a mouthful, drop a crumb, or have one extra nibble. I was determined to follow the plan down to the letter. With the results we'd seen early on, there was no way I wasn't going to give this my all.

It didn't take long for Will to develop a few favorite meals, especially because he was so willing. A typical breakfast for him would include an egg fried in oil, a cup of whipped cream, and three blueberries. For lunch he could have hotdogs or a cheeseburger but neither could be served on a bun or with any condiments. I had an awesome recipe for a keto-approved personal pizza that he really liked and was a great go-to on many occasions. I played around with pizza crust recipes for what seemed like an eternity. We settled on a combination of egg whites and Keto Cal powder (almost like a protein powder). I was constantly looking for new recipes to try to give Will as much variety as possible, given the laundry list of banned items and ingredients.

As Halloween rolled around again, Brian and I were ready. We packed the boys up into the wagon again and took them around the neighborhood to trick-or-treat. Then just like the year before, we set up the Halloween store at home, where Will was able to trade sweet treats for inedible trinkets and toys. That year, he was looking forward to shopping in the store fully aware that eating a single piece of candy could

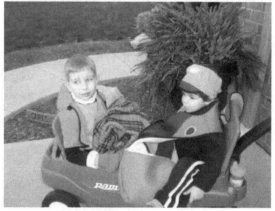

Another Halloween wagon ride!

ruin his diet and potentially induce a seizure. Nothing was going to derail Will from his diet and the fantastic way it was making him feel!

With the incredible improvement in Will's condition, we approached his 24-hour EEG the coming November with a sense of optimism I'd never dared to feel in his prior overnight observations. We'd gone in with the hope that we'd be able to wean Will off the Depakote. He'd been seizure-free since July 7th: four full months from that fateful case of Salmonella poisoning that kick-started his ketogenic diet. If this EEG came out clean, we planned to reduce his medication over the next two months until he was weaned off completely.

So, we packed up Will's grandpa pajamas again and prepared for another sleepover at Children's Hospital. It was the most stress-free, peaceful, hospital stay we'd ever had together. Will seemed to be feeling great the entire 24-hour period, despite being attached to the EEG machine. For the first time we were actually able to play some of the games and do some of the activities I'd always packed to pass the time. We enjoyed each other's company and bonded during the test. But the best part about it was the fact that I hadn't noticed a single seizure the entire time we were there. When Will's nurse practitioner called the following week to confirm that his EEG was clean, I felt like I could fly to the moon! They'd given us the green light to wean Will off his meds! It was the best possible news our family could be given. A miraculous gift that we cherished and celebrated that blessed holiday season. *Thank you, God!*

# CHAPTER 12
# MURPHY'S LAW: ANYTHING THAT CAN GO WRONG, WILL GO WRONG

The weeks passed by, and we were finally used to the ketogenic diet. I felt more comfortable and confident meal planning and had a good handle on the ingredients and supplies needed to comply. Will was cognizant of the impact that the diet was making. He felt healthy, normal. Or at least what he thought normal might feel like as he'd had so little experience with the sentiment. In any event, Will stuck to the plan without much complaint, which made it so much easier for everyone.

That's not to say it wasn't a challenge; it was an ever-present source of stress straining the very fabric of our family in ways I hadn't really anticipated. Will's entire world—our entire world—revolved around his diet. And because it wasn't simple to prepare his meals, we almost always ate at home. Who wants to bring a small piece of meat and three blueberries to a restaurant while everyone else is eating whatever they want or go to a party with a plastic container in tow and no leeway to taste anything else?

Our usually social family started to avoid all social situations. It was hard *having* to decline the countless invitations our family and friends extended to us during that time for picnics, parties, and barbecues. It was just too much stress for Will to handle, and unfortunately, elevated stress levels could trigger him to seize. Until Will was put on the ketogenic diet, I didn't fully appreciate just how much of what we do revolves around food.

Holidays, birthdays, and even playdates all seem to be centered around food. Not wanting to shun all celebrations, we began to time our arrivals and departures strategically to avoid the undue stress of bypassing a buffet. We'd show up for the activity (bowling, swimming, etc.) and sneak out before the pizza was passed or the cake was cut.

But social situations weren't the only source of our stress with the diet. At home, Will had a healthy and hungry, younger brother who craved the kinds of kid foods that we'd all but banished from our house. There was no reason why Blake couldn't have the fruit snacks, crackers, pretzels, and popsicles he wanted to snack on other than our desire to save Will from any added sorrow. I took to giving those forbidden foods to Blake on the sly, hiding with him in the laundry room to give him an apple out of plain sight. I can only imagine what Blake thought of it all: scarfing down secret snacks while surrounded by piles of dirty clothes! Playdates presented a similar problem as I couldn't very well offer Will's friends the same four macadamia nuts he was allowed for an afternoon snack, so it was easier to just forego hosting.

Inconvenience aside, time marched on toward the end of Will's time in kindergarten. It'd been a very good year considering everything that we'd experienced in preschool. We were fortunate our school district only offers half-day kindergarten: no lunch period, no snack break. On the few occasions when they were allowed to have a treat, the nurse would send a letter home so I could make a similar diet friendly version for Will. Thank goodness I'd perfected a mock cupcake; I swear it was the most useful recipe I had.

It certainly wasn't an overabundance of sugar that led to our little man's his first loose tooth. Will was growing up, but he wasn't ready to let that first tooth go. We showed up for his monthly neurology appointment and his nurse practitioner made a huge deal about his tooth as she pulled it out! This was a first: a *toothectomy* at the neurologist. Will was so pleased with himself the rest of the day, and he couldn't wait to put his first tooth under his pillow for the tooth fairy. Brian and I were thrilled to see Will so happy. His good mood was infectious, and Brian and I took a moment to just revel in his genuine joy.

The summer had become a scary season for us. For some unknown reason we couldn't seem to make it through June and July without some kind of medical drama. So, I wasn't all that surprised when we ended up in the emergency room promptly on June 1st. It was a warm day, and Will, Blake, and their friend Jack were playing together outside. Blake decided to get the hose out to cool everyone off, so he went out the back door, turned the

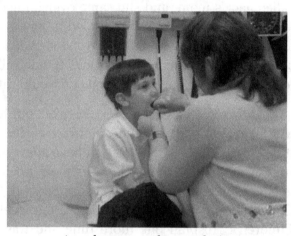

A toothectomy at the neurologist

hose on, and began spraying water everywhere. As (bad) luck would have it, Brian had stained the deck the week before, which made the treated wood planks very slippery when wet. When Will saw Blake outside with the hose, he excitedly threw open the patio door and he dashed out to join him. He took one step on the now slick deck and went flying. I was standing in the kitchen and watched the whole scene unfold in slow motion. Like a cartoon character slipping on a banana peel, Will's feet flew up over his body as his head hit the deck. I could not believe my eyes. My son, who'd been seizure free for the last 11 months had just jarred his precious brain in the fall. Trying to remain calm, I picked him up off the deck and carried him inside. He cried and whimpered for about five minutes before falling sound asleep. I knew that wasn't a good sign.

I was terrified that Will had suffered a concussion and the symptoms he displayed seemed to justify my fear. Thirty minutes after he'd fallen asleep, he woke up again, crying and holding his head. I immediately grabbed the phone and dialed the neurology department at Children's Hospital. After three attempts with no answer, I decided to get on the road. He needed to be checked out. I called Jack's mom, and she came over immediately and offered to keep an eye on Blake. It was a good thing too because I was having a hard time getting ahold of anyone else. Brian wasn't picking up, and I tried my mom a couple times to no avail, so I decided to just leave a message. Hopefully, someone would call me back!

I gathered the essentials: his blanket, our toothbrushes, and pjs. Most trips to Children's ended with us staying the night so I figured it'd be better to be prepared and have a few of our belongings with us. Bag in hand, I thanked Jack's mom for her help, kissed Blake goodbye, and off we went. I was torn between heading downtown to Children's and getting seen sooner at our local ER. I decided to call Children's Hospital one more time and was so excited to hear a human on the other end of the line! She told me to go to the closest ER, which was fine by me because it was only one mile away. As soon as I hung up with his doctor's office, my mom called me back. She couldn't believe what had happened either. Why was it always poor Will? Knowing how much I hated to be alone with Will at the hospital, my mom sprang into action, promising she'd meet me at the ER as soon as possible.

The ER staff at St. Clair Hospital was amazing. They took Will immediately to evaluate his condition and began to order tests. With a concussion suspected, they decided to send Will for a CT scan. You'd think that I'd be used to it by now, but watching them wheel my sweet Will away again in a hospital bed tore my heart out. I was so afraid of what they might find, and it was all I could do not to panic.

He fell asleep again before the scan, exhausted by the day's events and the trauma he'd sustained. He looked so peaceful laying there; it gave me hope he was going to be alright. Then right in the middle of the scan, Will suddenly awoke. He was understandably confused and terrified. He'd fallen asleep in a hospital bed and awakened inside of a scanner. They halted the test and waited for him to calm down before they tried again. Thankfully, Will was able to relax and the scan was completed successfully.

It didn't take long for the results to come back. I can hardly relay the utter relief and elation we felt when the scans were negative: no brain damage. Our prayers had been answered! Will was discharged that day with a minor concussion. We were thrilled that we didn't need to stay the night and headed home happily with a list of restrictions, care advice, and instructions to call his doctor the following day. We'd be seeing her soon anyway since he had a routine 24-hour EEG scheduled the very next week. Now, if we could just stay out of any hospital for the next seven days. It'd probably be a stretch, but one can always hope!

# CHAPTER 13
## MONKEYING AROUND

A week had passed since Will's slip and fall. We'd dodged a major bullet with the mild concussion he'd sustained but I was still reeling from the panic of what could have been. I was weary of allowing Will to participate in any activity that might aggravate his injury and make matters worse. So, when the end-of-year picnic rolled around at Will's school, Brian and I decided it'd be for the best if we all just took a raincheck and stayed home. Will was surprisingly upset. He'd missed the last few days of the school year due to his accident, and he didn't want to miss playing with his classmates one last time before everyone went their separate ways for summer vacation.

Despite my reluctance and reservations, I soon changed my mind. I mean, what could really go wrong at a two-hour, elementary school picnic? The day of the picnic, I prepared a ketogenic meal for Will that was as close as possible to what was being served. Hamburgers are standard picnic dinner fare and Will was fortunately allowed to have one. Though his comparatively tiny patty had to be carefully weighed, cooked in a sea of coconut oil, and served on a single leaf of lettuce: no bun, no cheese, no ketchup, or other condiments. Will was so happy to be surrounded by his friends that he didn't even seem to notice that his plate was different from anyone else's.

I wanted to be happy too, but I couldn't shake the persistent sense of impending doom that had taken root in my gut. I was paranoid, and I knew it, but it couldn't be helped. If something bad could happen to Will, it usually did, and the picnic was just rife with opportunities. Brian tried to ease my mind—to convince me that fresh air and friends were the best medicine—but I couldn't take my eyes off Will as I sat by the playground doing my best not to look as nervous as I felt. I doubt I was very convincing. As soon as I spotted him grab hold of the monkey bar glider, I got up and started to make my way toward him. I hadn't gone more than a few steps when I saw Will lose his grip and fall to the ground. I tried not to panic as I quickened my pace, thankful to at least see him stirring.

"See!" I yelled back at Brian, "I told you this was a bad idea!"

Will was already getting up but one look at the awkward bend in his arm and the way he was gripping his elbow was enough to tell me he'd gotten hurt. I glared at Brian as he tried in vain to reassure me.

"Will is fine," he said, "Kids fall off the monkey bars all the time. Relax!"

As if I could. I was worried and upset not only because Will had gotten hurt but because we put him in a situation to do so. Why hadn't I trusted my instincts and stuck with our original decision to skip the picnic? Why did the school have such old, unsafe equipment? Why did it always have to be Will that got hurt? Why? Why? Why?

Before I could spiral out of control, a couple of our amazing neighbors rushed over to help. One of them, a physical therapist, looked at Will's elbow, turning his little arm gently in his hands. After he evaluated it, he called over another neighbor who happens to be a doctor for her opinion. She agreed that we should err on the side of caution and take Will in for an x-ray. It was 8 p.m. on a Friday night, and we had a decision to make: take Will to Urgent Care down the street or head to the ER? Urgent Care was closer, but they were also set to close soon. At the doctor's urging, we decided to try to make it to Urgent Care before they locked up for the night. I was beside myself as we packed up our things and raced to the car, torn between wanting to scream or cry and doing neither for the sake of our sons. It was ironic, to say the least, that the hospital medevac helicopter was just touching down on the field by the school—as it did every year—as we sped away in search of Urgent Care. I glanced at the whirring blades as they slowed in the air, wishing like hell we could just hop inside and get the medical attention Will needed right then. Instead, we all buckled up, sped down the street, and made it to Urgent Care in record time.

The staff there was wonderful, taking us back as soon as we'd arrived to x-ray Will's arm. The doctor read the film and determined the x-ray was inconclusive. So, they gave Will a sling and an adorable, little teddy bear and told us to follow up with an orthopedic doctor on Monday. As we poured ourselves back into the car for the short ride home, Will was still in pain, and I was completely exhausted. We were weary and tired, worn down by the seemingly endless stream of unfortunate events that followed our oldest son like a singularly determined, dark cartoon cloud. Meanwhile, our youngest son just went along for the ride, used to the doctoring Will endured and feeling understandably slighted. He eyed Will's teddy bear with envy and asked, "Why does Will always get prizes?" He was too young then to realize that Will wasn't the lucky one.

The weekend seemed to drag by extra slowly as we waited for Monday and the appointment with the orthopedic doctor to arrive. When it finally did, I half expected my car to navigate to the hospital by itself after the number of trips we'd made there over the years. Once inside though, we found ourselves on unfamiliar ground as we headed to the unexplored orthopedic wing. The line of patients waiting to be x-rayed was long and the injuries were varied, but almost all had one thing in common: the cause of the injury. A doctor came out to address the crowd, asking by a show of hands, which patients there had sustained their injuries on a trampoline or monkey bars. I was stunned to see nine of the ten kids waiting in line raise their hands! It was unreal. We will NEVER get a trampoline.

When it was our turn to meet with the doctor, he admitted that he couldn't find much damage but thought it best to put Will in a full arm cast. What a perfect way for our sweet six-year-old to start his summer vacation—a concussion, a cast, and a super strict diet! He wouldn't be able to write, eat, play sports, swim, play video games, or watch too much TV. It was going to be a long, few months.

As we left the appointment with Will's right arm in a full cast, we decided to break our post-hospital tradition of visiting the castle park. We were both anxious to get back home since we knew we'd be heading back to the hospital in just another week. Will's 24-hour EEG had been scheduled four months ago, and although we weren't necessarily looking forward to another night in the hospital, we weren't about to wait another day. We were dying to know how his brain was doing. It had been almost one full year on the ketogenic diet and that test would reveal the exact impact our efforts had on his brain. We could hardly wait to get the results!

I did have some concerns that Will's recent concussion might affect his results, but not enough to deter us from having the test as scheduled. I found myself reflecting as I went through the motions of once again packing our overnight bags. We'd had our share of scares, trauma, and more visits to the ER than I ever imagined in my lifetime before Will had been born. And yet, we were some of the lucky ones. We always got to go home, always had some semblance of a normal life between the valleys. Many of the other families we saw huddled in the waiting rooms and wandering down the halls of Children's weren't so lucky.

It broke my heart every time I watched Will seize and suffer. I'd have given anything to take his place, but we never gave up hope. The ketogenic diet was taxing and precise, taking hours to track down and prepare the ingredients, but we did it with an unwavering faith and tenacity. We did it because it made a difference. It was as if we had pressed a "reset" button rebooting Will's brain and chasing the *bad guys* away ... hopefully for good. This crucial test would tell us for sure.

The week between Will's fall at the picnic and his overnight EEG went by far too slowly. We were anxious to get there and relieved when the day finally arrived. Rather than taking us to a closet-size room where the scent from the adhesives would make our heads spin, the EEG tech kindly came to our room and started the tedious task of placing the electrodes all over Will's head. It was nice to have a little more breathing room—literally. We passed the time watching movies and chatting before Will fell asleep. I hadn't noticed him having a single seizure in the 24-hour period that he was connected, and we could only hope his results would show the same.

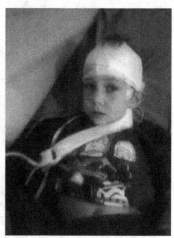

Will with a concussion, a broken arm, and an EEG.

The next morning, we packed up and waited for our discharge papers. Will was excited to get home, and I was too. On our way to the parking garage, we passed the gift shop, and I was just waiting for Will to ask for a prize. Instead, he spied an extra-large mylar Mickey Mouse balloon that Blake would go nuts over. After a night in the hospital, Will wanted to buy Blake a gift! "Yes," I said, "the answer is yes, we can buy that for your little brother."

We left the hospital, thankful for a blissfully boring stay, and headed back home to wait for the results. EEGs typically take a week or two to be read and reported, so imagine my surprise when we received a call from Will's nurse practitioner the very next day. She was ecstatic as she shared the findings—his EEG was *normal!* I was so stunned I couldn't even speak. I broke down and started to sob, catching Will's attention.

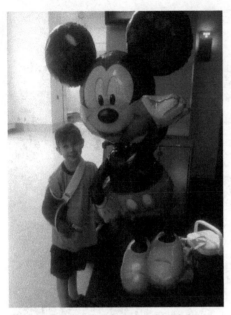

A giant Mickey balloon for Blake

He ran over to me immediately and said, "Oh no, mommy. What did the doctor tell you?" The nurse practitioner had overheard him and got emotional as well.

We'd been through so many bad results; it was surreal to hear the words we'd hoped and prayed about for years. Will was finally seizure free! The tears kept rolling down my cheeks as I listened to the next steps: no more medicine and no more special meals. It was a miracle that had all been made possible by an unexpected case of Salmonella poisoning. The ketogenic diet had scared the monsters away and brought our son back. For that, we'll be forever grateful.

# CHAPTER 14
## PARTY TIME

Our house was filled with happiness and our hearts were filled with gratitude. Our prayers had been answered, and we could hardly wait to celebrate. I hate to admit that it took a few days for the news to sink in. To believe—without a shadow of doubt—that Will had a clean bill of health. After the long and difficult rollercoaster ride we'd all been on since his initial diagnosis, no one could blame me for being a bit hesitant to accept this miraculous gift. Still, I'd heard the results with my own ears and seen them myself with my own two eyes just days after he'd started the diet. Will's seizures were gone, and it was time to party!

The final day of Will's ketogenic diet arrived and it's hard to say who was more excited. We invited his best buddy, Jack, and his family over to share in this milestone. I was downright giddy as I prepared his last ketogenic meal. My days of measuring and weighing every bite would soon be a distant memory. It was a beautiful night, and we decided to grill out. I filled Will's plate with one hot dog, a hamburger, a dollop of whipped cream, and a few pieces of broccoli that had been drenched in butter. Will ate his *last supper* with a smile on his face, knowing full well that the best was yet to come. Brian and I had decided to let Will have his first real dessert in over two years—a scoop of Sarris's chocolate chip cookie dough ice cream—a treat from a local chocolate factory. Real ice cream! Will could hardly contain himself! It was a wonderful moment with our family and dear friends, who'd been so incredibly supportive throughout this whole journey. We all gathered around and watched with bated breath as Will lifted the first spoonful to his mouth. I couldn't stop the tears that filled my eyes as he savored the treat he'd been denied for so long. Yes, I cried as I watched my six-year-old eat a scoop of ice cream. It was a moment I will never forget.

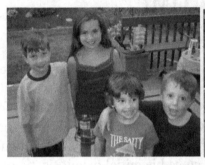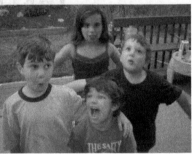

An ice cream party with neighbors

The following morning, Will woke up at 6 a.m. and came bounding into our bedroom. He was nearly vibrating with enthusiasm as he declared with a smile, "Watch out food, here I come!" It felt a bit like Christmas morning as Brian and I hopped out of bed to follow Will into the kitchen, but instead of eyeing a pile of presents and trying to decide which one to open first, Will contemplated which culinary delight he wanted to sample first. I was surprised to see him grab a banana. How funny is that? He couldn't wait to eat a whole banana. Not an ounce or a few measly slices, but the whole thing. Having started off with a healthy snack, Will was ready for the good stuff. He wanted a cinnamon roll. I hesitated for a moment, terrified of what all that sugar might do to his brain, but ultimately, we let him have it. We needed to have faith that his brain would be OK and that his tiny body would continue to fight to stay well. I confess I might've watched him like a hawk for a few hours after he ate it. I was relieved to see that he'd handled it just fine.

Feeling assured that everything was going to be fine, we all got back to the business of living life to the fullest and cherishing every healthy moment. We also felt the need to celebrate our good fortune at home with our wonderful family and the countless childhood, high school, and college friends, teammates, co-workers, and neighbors who'd all been there offering their incredible love and support throughout this whole saga.

What better way to celebrate with such a big group than with a party at our house? We wanted to make up for all the birthday parties and holidays we'd missed because of Will's restrictions, but this time, nothing would be off limits. We wanted to involve Will in planning the party and let him decide the theme and the menu. He decided we should call it the *Off the Diet!* party, and we loved the idea.

For the last two years, I'd done my best to mimic some of Will's favorite foods using the limited ingredients I had at my disposal. *Tried* being the operative word as there was really no way I could ever make any of his meals look or taste like the real foods he was forbidden to have. So, I guess I shouldn't have been shocked at all when Will wrote *real* in front of every item he'd wanted to serve at the party: *real* pizza, *real* cupcakes, *real* candy, and the list continued. The poor kid just wanted *real* food and we were going to give it to him—plenty of it. I felt compelled to include a warning to our guests on the invitations that this would not be a typical party at the Simmons' house and to be ready to indulge.

But the party was about more than just an abundance of junk food. This was our chance to finally relax and catch up with our family and friends, to treat them to a fun afternoon, and thank them for their love and support. We tried to transform our yard into a carnival-like atmosphere. We hired a balloon artist and set up games in the yard with prizes for all the kids. It was so great to see everyone smiling and laughing and just having a good time, especially Will.

At one point in the evening, my dad made sure everyone had a fresh drink before he offered a toast. As soon as he opened his mouth, tears started to run down my face (shocker!). First, he congratulated Will, expressing his indescribable joy for his grandson's good health. Then he turned to Brian and I and raised his glass to thank us for never giving up the fight, for doing everything in our power to help Will get better. Finally, he turned to our good friends and neighbors to thank them all for being there for our family—in good times and bad. He said it was an honor to be there celebrating with us, but it was our little family of four that felt honored to be surrounded by so many amazing, caring, incredible people. By the time my dad had finished his toast, there wasn't a dry eye to be found. Everyone had been moved to tears; tears of joy for Will and the bright future that lay ahead of him. It was one of the happiest days of my life.

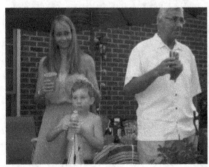 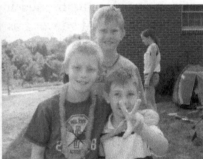

Poppy's toast at the *Off the Diet!* Party (left), Having a blast with Nick and Luke (right)

When things are going well, it's easy to find happiness ... even in circumstances that might otherwise be upsetting. A week after the party, I found myself in one of those very situations—laughing uncontrollably when I should've been livid instead. It was a lazy Sunday morning and I'd been catching up with a long-distance friend on the phone. About 20 minutes into our conversation, it dawned on me that something was amiss. It was suspiciously peaceful and quiet in the house: too quiet. Most days, I'd be lucky to spend five minutes on a call, let alone 20, and I remember telling my friend, "The boys are actually getting along right now, I hear them giggling in Will's bedroom. How sweet!"

How *sweet* it was for them indeed! While I was preoccupied on the phone, the boys had decided to form their very own candy club! Somehow Blake had found the candy stash and snuck it into Will's bedroom. Then, while I chatted away, the two of them proceeded to develop and execute the rules of this new club: *eat lots of candy!*

When I finally hung up, I found them both heading down the stairs. Blake had his blanket draped over the candy container, which was suspicious to say the least.

Then Will asked, "Mommy, when is dinner?"

I looked at my watch. It was 11:20 a.m. "Not for a long time," I replied. "Why?"

Will looked a little sheepish as he answered, "I hope you won't be mad, but I think we spoiled our dinner." I had just started to put the pieces together when he added, "I think you should check my garbage can!"

I could barely contain the smile on my face: the honesty ... I loved it!

I was understandably intrigued by then and turned straightaway to head to Will's room. When I arrived and looked in the garbage can, I was shocked to find it filled to the brim with candy wrappers. Specifically, I found the following:

- A Sarris candy bar wrapper
- A Hershey's chocolate bar wrapper
- Two M&M wrappers
- A Swedish Fish wrapper
- A Goldfish wrapper
- Two fruit snack wrappers

Instead of being angry or upset as I might've been under different circumstances, I couldn't help but laugh.

It was official, the Candy Club had been created and Will and Blake were the first members! Blake was so proud. "We actually talked to each other and shared candy. It was so much fun, Mom!" he bragged.

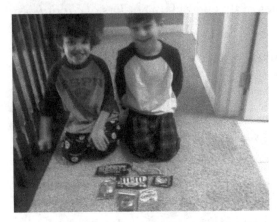

The Candy Club

If this had happened a year ago, an innocent act of brotherly bonding would have meant serious medical consequences for Will. We would have been on our way to Children's Hospital and likely been witness to a slew of sugar-induced seizures. But that was then, and this was now. I wasn't worried or angry about the gluttonous binge. The worst thing that would likely happen was an upset tummy or maybe the makings of a cavity. I was happy and relieved. They were just kids being kids, and there was no way I could be mad about that.

That's not to say we condoned their behavior and allowed them to eat whatever they wanted, whenever they wished. After those initial days, we settled back into a normal eating routine with a diet comprised of a healthy mix of proteins, carbohydrates, fresh fruits, vegetables, and occasional goodies and treats. Will was feeling fine, but we still needed to attend one last ketogenic clinic appointment. This would be the best one ever because it would be our last: no blood work, no testing, and no poking or prodding. Even though we were happy that we wouldn't be going back, we were sure going to miss the amazing team of doctors, nurses, dieticians, and techs.

They'd all helped Will tremendously along his journey. It had been 16 months since his last recorded seizure and four months since he'd stopped the ketogenic diet. He was feeling good, and so were we. He's a tough kid and we were (and are still) so proud of how he handled his hardships. Goodbye you ugly monsters, please don't mess with Will ever again!

Luckily, in the months that followed, Will stayed healthy, and life was status quo. We enjoyed the lack of drama and the time off from the hospital. We got back to the basics of being a young, average American family, and it felt so good. Will was going on 20 months of being hospital free, medication free, diet free and—most importantly—seizure free, and that was a milestone worth celebrating.

# CHAPTER 15
# THE CRUISE

After all we'd been through, we decided that we needed and had earned a vacation. More than just a getaway, we wanted to celebrate! We went back and forth about where to go and what to do. In the end, we decided to go on a Disney cruise. Both boys were into boats and airplanes, so we figured they'd be excited about flying to Florida and boarding a gigantic cruise ship. And if those two things weren't exciting enough, then the promise of *24/7, all-you-can-eat dining* would certainly seal the deal. Will could hardly wait to get on board and dig in!

The kids were excited to see our plans come together as we got passports, made packing lists, and purchased a few new items just for the trip. After months of waiting, the day had finally arrived, and we were ready to set sail. Watch out Bahamas, here we come!

Blake had never been on an airplane before, and his excitement was palpable and contagious. There's something incredibly enchanting about watching your children experience things for the first time: to see the world through their eyes for a moment and share in their thrill of the unknown. Their sense of genuine awe is infectious. The flight was pleasant and uneventful, and we were all excited to touch down in Florida.

We decided to arrive a day before the cruise to avoid any hassle with how common flight delays and cancelations have become. With our baggage in tow, we checked into a hotel down the street from the port. The boys both love hotels and could hardly wait to get their swimsuits on and head for the pool. We let them swim and play right up until dinner time—we were on vacation and loving it!

The next morning, we sealed up our bags and headed to the port. Will and Blake were both overwhelmed by the enormous size of the ship. They couldn't believe we would be living on it for the next five days! As we waited patiently in line to check in for the cruise, I noticed that Will looked a little unsteady. I tried my best to ignore it and shake the bad thoughts out of my head. Will was fine. Everything was fine. But not more than ten minutes later, I watched in horror as Will slipped and fell, hitting his head on the hard concrete floor. I bolted over and picked him up off the floor as if he'd just had a seizure. I'm sure the people who'd witnessed his fall must've thought I was overreacting, but the truth was I couldn't help myself. I was then and always will be an overprotective, nervous mom, and I'm sure that I was more upset than Will as he dusted himself off. Still, I was relieved to see he hadn't hurt himself too badly. No major cuts or bruises—except to his ego (maybe)— that needed medical attention. In fact, the whole thing was soon forgotten the moment we boarded the ship. The interiors of these grandiose cruise ships are truly spectacular, and we were all in awe of the scale and splendor as we made our way through the common areas.

When we got to our cabin, Will was happy to see that the lifeboats were one level below us. He had read a book about the Titanic and was a little worried about whether our ship had enough lifeboats for everyone on board. He cracks me up sometimes! He's such an old soul—so endearing and sweet. He also wanted to know if our ship was as big as the Titanic. Once we assured him that yes, our ship was both bigger than the Titanic and fully equipped with enough lifeboats, I could see his apprehension melt away. It was time to enjoy our vacation.

The check-in and boarding process took most of the morning, and by the time we got everything settled in our room, we were all starving. We all but ran straight to the welcome lunch which is typically a king-size buffet. Will's eyes nearly popped out of his head as he scanned the seemingly endless bins of food. He grabbed a plate and piled it up high before coming to find us at our table. Brian and I watched with glee as Will sat down to enjoy his feast. He ate and ate and ate until, after two full plates, he was finally done. We were beaming with pride and happiness as Will slumped down in his seat, full and sated in ways he couldn't imagine not so long ago. It's a strange thing getting teary eyed while watching your child enjoy his food, but after he'd been denied such simple pleasures for so long, it really was a joyous occasion. I'm sure the people who were sitting around us were

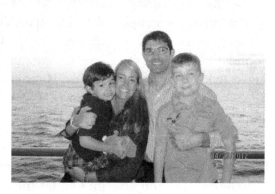

Our celebratory cruise

probably confused as to why Brian and I would be so proud of Will's gluttonous eating, but in that moment, we might as well have been the only people on board. It was a good moment. It felt like this trip was the final chapter of Will's long, arduous story. We'd lived the nightmare, we'd put it to bed, and this cruise was our way of putting it all behind us and moving on. We were finally able to do all the things that we used to avoid because of his epilepsy and diet. It felt wonderful!

As we sat there together with the ocean waves rippling outside and the sun shining brightly in the sky, I caught myself daydreaming about how lucky we were to finally be on the other side of our health struggles. It had been such a long time coming, filled with more dark days than I'd like to admit; days when I wondered if we'd ever see an end to Will's suffering. And yet, there we were, free at last. As I snapped out of my reverie, something caught my eye and stole my breath simultaneously: a Make-a-Wish® button. A family had been passing by our table, each one of them wearing a Make-a-Wish t-shirt. I couldn't help the overwhelming sadness I felt when a little boy—this family's son, brother, nephew, grandson—walked by with a button pinned to his chest that read, "I'm Making My Wish."

Seeing that family took me back to one of Will's specialist appointments a couple of years ago. The doctor mentioned in passing that Will's condition qualified for the Make-a-Wish Foundation. I couldn't believe my ears or make sense of what she'd suggested. Will was *not* that sick. He couldn't be. He wouldn't be.

I politely declined the doctor's offer and said we'd rather save those wishes for families who were truly in need. She knew we were serious about our fight and determined to win, so she never brought it up again. When faced with adversity, you really only have two choices: (1) You give up and let the chips fall where they may, or (2) You decide to fight and win. We'd made our decision early on—no matter what obstacles we faced or how many crushing setbacks and disappointments we weathered; nothing would stop us.

I closed my eyes and said a prayer for this family that was clearly still in the throes of a serious illness. I willed them the same strength of conviction we'd held fast to—to keep on fighting and never give up. I wanted so badly to reach out and hug them, to hear their story and wish them well. But the words got stuck in my throat and I couldn't even find the courage to say hello. I was able to smile with my lips pressed tightly together as I fought back the tears that were stinging my eyes. I had to turn away before I completely lost it. I wiped my eyes on my napkin before anyone could notice and took a deep breath. We were there to celebrate Will's good health and I didn't want to tarnish that.

That wasn't the only button we saw during our trip. Many families were there fulfilling their wishes. Every time I saw one of these families, I said a little prayer of thanks for our good fortune, while also saying a prayer of hope for the others still caught in the fight. After all, tons of hugs, lots of hope, and many prayers had helped us through our toughest times, and now we wanted to pay it forward. So, I say to all, "Have hope, pray often, and hug more!"

# CHAPTER 16
# NOT-SO-SMOOTH SAILING

Lounging on a deck chair next to Brian, with my face in the sun, the wind in my hair, and the kids in the pool, I took a deep breath and savored the moment. No meds, no scales, no blood work, no urine analysis strips ... and no worries. Someone could've caught me humming "Hakuna Matata" while I soaked up the sun. It was a Disney cruise, after all.

The cruise had been going well. The boys loved the ship and thought our state room was super cool because their beds folded down from the wall. They looked forward to seeing what kind of funny towel animals our housekeeper would make and leave in the room each day. The food was delicious, and Will especially enjoyed the all-you-can-eat buffet. Brian and I were having a good time too. Or at least I was until I thought I'd witnessed Will having two staring spells (absence seizures). I didn't want to believe it. So, I convinced myself that I was crazy, a hypochondriac, or just plain old seeing things. I didn't mention anything to Brian or the boys while we were on the boat, though I'm sure they could tell something with me was off. I've always worn my heart on my sleeve, so despite my glued-on smile, I couldn't completely mask my concern. After we returned home, it wasn't long before I was sure I noticed a couple more. Then one day my mom witnessed one, another day Brian had as well. We all knew what was happening, but no one wanted to acknowledge it.

We were in denial. Will, most of all. He became very defensive every time I asked if he was alright. He'd huff his annoyance and say, "Mom that was not a seizure!" The irony in his staunch refusal was that Will never could tell when he'd had a seizure. He had no memory or awareness of any of the seizures he'd ever experienced.

Still, he was angry at us all the same for so much as suggesting that he had. I was thankful that he'd only been experiencing absence seizures (formerly known as petit mal seizures). Lasting for approximately 15-30 seconds, these brief spells are often mistaken as daydreaming. But I'd been around this block before, and I knew when he was having a seizure. Sometimes his eyelids fluttered, and his eyes rolled up and back, but more often than not he'd just stare off into space as a little monster in his brain flipped some kind of switch—off, on, off, on—without any rhyme or reason.

At first, I told myself, Be happy; it's only the occasional absence seizure. Before the ketogenic diet, he'd been having multiple types and hundreds of them a day at that. I tried to convince myself that it wasn't too bad, that maybe if we just closed our eyes and made a wish, the seizures would just stop and go away. It became apparent after a couple weeks we could no longer ignore what was happening to Will. The bad guys were back, and it was time to take action.

I contacted his first-grade teacher to see if she had noticed anything different about Will in class. She said that he'd been complaining of headaches on a regular basis and asked to go to the nurse often. We too noticed that he seemed to be having a lot of headaches, so I added that to our list to talk with his neurologist about.

Luckily there was only one week of school left. It would be much easier to monitor Will over the summer and try to figure out what was going on. Once again, I was grateful to be able to stay at home full-time. I can't imagine what I would've done or what would've happened if I was unable to be at home. We'd been down this road before, and I knew it was going to take my full time and attention to hunt down the answers we needed to determine an appropriate treatment plan.

I knew to achieve either of those goals that I needed to call Will's neurologist. The same one who'd discharged Will and handed me Will's file last November. It pained me to have to make that call. I had sincerely hoped I'd never need their services again. After all, Will had grown out of his epilepsy! But no matter how hard I prayed or wished them away; his seizures were back, and the battle was on again. It was time to get geared up and get back in the fight.

Will's incredible nurse practitioner was shocked to hear my voice. She was so disappointed to learn that Will had relapsed. I booked an appointment and broke the news to Will that we had to go back to Children's Hospital to talk with his neurologist again. I thought I'd learned my lesson early on about promises and knowing better than to make them. I promised Will we were done with the neurology department when we were released last fall, and now we had to head back. Our journey with epilepsy wasn't over, and Will wasn't ready to go back. He was angry and in denial, and I couldn't blame him; no one could. "Why me?" he asked. "Doesn't God love me? I prayed for my seizures to go away." It broke my heart when he asked those questions, especially when I had no answers to give.

I knew that Will needed me to be resilient and stoic—a pillar of strength—even as I felt like my world was crumbling down around me. I couldn't allow myself to dwell on how unfair life could be or to feel as Will did in the wake of this terrible turn of events: hopeless, angry, defeated, and depressed. So, I had a good cry when no one was looking, straightened my shoulders, took a deep breath, and rolled up my sleeves. We needed to fight these monsters again, and I didn't want to waste another minute.

In addition to putting on a brave face, I also needed to watch what I said in front of Will. Whenever he'd overhear me talking to my mom or mother in-law about his seizures, he'd get very upset and defensive. I turned to my moms, as I always did, to glean their knowledge as nurses, their strength as loving parents, and their unwavering support as grandmothers. But Will was no longer a naïve four-year-old. He was a savvy seven-year-old who understood what we were talking about and what was at stake—his good health and happiness. He knew that his brief stint of *normalcy* was nearing its end. All the things he thought were behind him were once again staring him in the face: more doctors, more tests, more seizures, and more uncertainty.

I made the calls that needed to be made to get the ball rolling again. The first order of business before we could schedule his neurology appointment was to have an EEG. The doctors wanted to see what was happening in his brain, and they wanted a new baseline of data before they saw him at the hospital. We scheduled the EEG for the end of May, and when the day rolled around, we decided at the last minute to cancel it. Will had three weeks of school left, and we agreed that the test could wait until summer break. If it seems like we were dragging our feet, we were. We knew where we were ultimately headed ... back to the ketogenic diet, and that was a daunting prospect that we just weren't ready to face.

Unfortunately, over that span of time, things were not getting any better. His seizures were becoming more frequent but were still a far cry from the number he'd had in the past. Prior to the ketogenic diet, he was experiencing more than 50 seizures a day. So, the 10 to 15 that he'd been having since we'd returned from the cruise seemed oddly *doable*.

Late spring is a busy time of year for us. From baseball games to end-of-school-year parties, we were doing everything we could to distract ourselves from the inevitable. I guess we needed a wake-up call and that's exactly what we got. Two days after school let out, Will woke up with a fever and a headache. Most people would not hope and pray that their child had contracted a case of strep throat, but that's exactly what we hoped might be behind Will's symptoms. Strep is easily diagnosed and readily treated with a course of antibiotics, but things have never been so simple with Will. Why would this be any different?

As usual, at the same time Will started feeling ill, Brian and I had plans for the weekend that had been scheduled months before. We had planned a Saturday afternoon field trip with some of our neighbors to a local vineyard. We had a driver lined up and had offered to have an after party at our house that evening. I was about to cancel when my mom insisted on taking the kids and promised to keep a watchful eye on Will. By the time she picked them up, his fever was gone, and he seemed to be feeling fine. I'm a firm believer that wine makes everything better, so off we went to the wine tasting! We had a great time, of course, and I was relieved when my mom dropped the kids off and said that Will had been fine while we were out. Unfortunately, his fever had returned that evening, and he said he felt achy all over.

By the next day, Will was having trouble walking. He said his legs hurt so badly he couldn't make it to the bathroom. His fever hadn't let up and he was extremely lethargic. I was nervous, as usual, and decided to call his pediatrician. They wanted to see him right away since they knew his seizures always got worse whenever he had a fever. It's regrettably common in kids with epilepsy. True to form, Will started having a ton of seizures and then developed a rash on his face. He has sensitive skin and is prone to rashes, but they always manage to freak me out. The pediatrician spent a couple minutes examining Will before he admitted that he wasn't sure exactly what was going on. He recommended we head to the Children's Hospital ER immediately and said he would call ahead for us, so they'd be ready when we arrived.

Although I'd hoped these days were behind us, at least I knew exactly what needed to happen. I had to find a place for poor little Blake to go while we were gone; I needed to pack an overnight bag for me and Will; and I needed to grab his favorite blanket! Within ten minutes, we were on our way to Children's. I was used to the drive and knew some back ways to avoid traffic and detours, but I was feeling a little uneasy. He was really sick, and I was alone and terrified of what they were going to tell me this time.

The ER doctor contacted the neurology department, and they started to go back and forth trying to diagnose this latest funk. I heard them mention meningitis, encephalitis, a spinal tap; I was panicking, and Will was laying on the hospital bed seizing. My head was spinning, and all I could think was *This isn't fair, this isn't fair, this isn't fair!* I wanted to wave a magic wand and switch places with my seven-year-old. How much more could his sweet little body handle?

I managed to get my act together long enough to ask the doctors

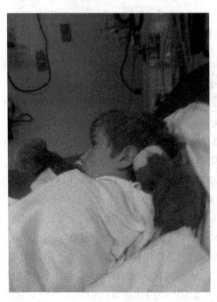

Another hospital visit

to please give him some fluids. They hooked him up to the IV, and 20 minutes later he started to perk up a little. He still had a rash all over his cheeks, and his fever persisted, but the scariest part of all was his ongoing inability to walk. His legs weren't strong enough to hold up his body. He weighed 65 pounds at the time and was getting too big for me to pick up and carry around. And I wonder why my back hurts sometimes!

Over the next few hours, many people popped in to review Will's case—residents, interns, students, nurses—but no one had any answers. I needed someone to help us, and I needed them immediately. I decided to text a dear friend and neighbor who worked as an oncology nurse at the hospital.

My message read, *Are you here today? Will and I are in the ER.*

Three minutes later, she walked into Will's room. It was so wonderful to see a familiar face and get a much-needed hug from a dear friend to calm my frazzled nerves. It turned out she was in the elevator on her way to lunch when she received my message. What a coincidence, she was there and available right when I needed her. She comforted Will and put my mind at ease, giving me the reassurance that I so desperately needed.

The nurse came in a short time later to do some blood work. Will was so used to giving his blood up for testing, he didn't even flinch. He casually asked how many vials she needed as he offered his arm. He is such a trooper! Then it was time to watch and wait. His blood was being tested and his IV drip was keeping him hydrated. I was thankful to see that Will seemed to be feeling a little better. Four hours later, we received his diagnosis. They said he was fighting a virus and discharged him on the spot to rest and recover at home. I was so relieved it wasn't meningitis or encephalitis. At the same time, I was a little disappointed that it wasn't more a definitive diagnosis like a positive strep culture.

I could only pray that this virus was responsible for his recurring seizures and that once it left him alone, it would take the seizures with it too ... for good this time. Before we were discharged from the ER, we finally relented and scheduled the EEG we'd been trying to avoid. We needed to track his seizure activity and get a clear picture of just how many he was actually having.

Over the next few days, his symptoms subsided. The rash began to fade as did the debilitating joint pain and ongoing fever. The seizures, unfortunately, continued to occur, which was beyond demoralizing. At least Will could get some satisfaction in the knowledge that his upcoming EEG would only take 40 minutes to complete. Woo-hoo! The last couple he'd had lasted between 24–96 hours!

Will's first week of summer vacation was a real bummer, but he was starting to regain some energy and was looking a lot more like himself. I was so relieved that he was feeling better, but, like Will, I wasn't really looking forward to the EEG. I really didn't need it to confirm what I already knew and begrudgingly accepted; Will's seizures were back, and we were pissed.

# CHAPTER 17
## CONFIRMATION

It was time to face the facts, Will's epilepsy was back after almost two years of freedom. Despite the obvious signs, we needed to confirm our fears with an EEG. Will was surprisingly calm about going for this test. He said he was really looking forward to getting his reward afterward. I love children and their wonderful outlook on life. Will was ready to conquer this thing and get to the nearest toy store. Whatever it takes! I never thought I'd be the kind of parent who would bribe their kids, but just like Mary Poppins sang, "A spoonful of sugar helps the medicine go down." So, if the promise of a prize made continual poking, prodding, and testing more palatable, then so be it. I have zero guilt, zero regrets.

My mom had dropped us off and took Blake to the park during the EEG. As we sat in the waiting room, I witnessed two absence seizures. I remember thinking it wasn't even necessary to do this test, but we were there, and I knew his doctor needed confirmation. Luckily, Will's favorite EEG tech was on staff that day. As he placed the electrodes on Will's head, Will proceeded to have two more seizures. I swear he had more seizures when we are at any type of doctor's office or hospital. I can't say if it was stress and anxiety or the lighting in the room or simply that he knew what he was supposed to do. I've heard of children who are the opposite of Will—unable to have seizures captured on EEGs but fall into them after they've been disconnected—like some form of stage fright or performance anxiety. Will has never had that problem, which I guess is a good thing. He's always been a people pleaser and a rule follower who hates to disappoint, and when it came time to be tested, he never did.

As soon as all the electrodes were secure and the machine was turned on, Will was seizing within the first minute. The tech recorded six additional seizures in the first ten minutes and confirmed to me that Will's epilepsy was back for sure. Our worst nightmare had returned. We thought we'd said our goodbyes to his seizures and truly believed he grew out of it. I was overwhelmed with sadness and anger. It just wasn't fair, and it didn't make sense. The ketogenic diet had cured him!

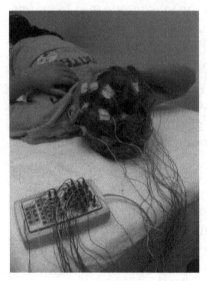

EEG time ... again

My thoughts were a blur, and I was unable to speak when the tech announced, "Well, we got all the information we needed. I captured multiple seizures. Will's neurologist will call you as soon as possible to discuss the treatment plan."

Even though I wasn't surprised by the outcome, I was still devastated. As we wandered through the hospital halls and made our way out of the building, I felt like a zombie: numb, listless, and shocked by the validation of my greatest fear.

My mom must've seen the devastation written on my face as we approached the car.

She took one look at me and asked, "How bad?"

I answered, "Worse than we thought."

I mean I knew Will had been seizing but the tech had recorded more in that short span of time than I'd witnessed up to that point. That's the tough thing about seizures in general, some are painfully obvious while others are so subtle if you blinked, you'd miss them. I was thankful that Will appeared to be experiencing mostly absence seizures (staring spells and eye flutters) and not tonic-conic seizures (convulsing type). Obviously, I'd rather he have no seizures at all, but at least this variety felt more manageable.

The timing of these test results turned out to be horrible. I was scheduled to leave on a flight later that day for a long weekend away with neighborhood friends. I guess there's never a good time to deal with bad news or health issues, but I seemed to find myself in this position once a year ... and it sucked. This time, I was heading to Chicago for one of my closest friend's 40th birthday celebration: a weekend long extravaganza in Chicago that had been in the works for months. I began to beat myself up about going and talked it over with my mom the whole way home. She convinced me that I should go and that nothing had really changed from earlier that day. The only difference being that now we had definitive confirmation of what we already knew. And when I talked with Brian, he agreed that I should go.

So, I quickly made a few phone calls, grabbed my suitcase, kissed the kids, and I was off to the airport with my girlfriends. My mom had the boys until Brian got home from work, so they were in heaven ... they always love some Nonny time! She'd be building forts and telling stories and spoiling them rotten. It was reassuring to know that they'd be in good hands and having a great time. It definitely eased the guilt I was feeling.

I took a deep breath and tried to switch gears into fun girl's weekend mode, but it was tough. My neighborhood gang of friends are beyond great. They're understanding, compassionate, and empathetic women. Almost all of them have experienced difficult health situations in their own families as well. Sometimes we'd commiserate and discuss how it must've been fate for us all to be friends. I smiled and thought how lucky I am to have these ladies in my life. A moment later, the phone rang.

It was the nurse practitioner from the neurology department. She received the EEG results and was calling to discuss our options. First, she reiterated the sadness that she shared with us on Will's relapse. She'd been so happy to discharge us and hand me Will's file just eight short months ago. She had hoped, as we all did, for a miraculous success story. I took a deep breath and prepared myself for a list of options I didn't even want to hear. She suggested trying a medication called Zarontin, one of the few that Will hadn't tried. I struggled with the suggestion because we *hate* drugs and the awful side effects they'd always had on him. She also said that we could try the ketogenic diet again knowing how well it worked for us.

As much as we were keen on the diet the first time around, I was not excited about this option again. Will was finally thriving and found so much comfort in eating normal food. He'd been deprived of it for two years and was truly enjoying every bite since he'd come off the diet. Toward the end, I could tell he felt embarrassed by his *special* food, and he'd been looking forward to starting second grade diet, drug, and seizure free. I knew Will would be devastated to learn that none of his hopes would likely come to pass. I also knew that now was not the time to make a decision.

I thanked the neurologist and told her we'd take the weekend to weigh our options and that I'd call her on Monday with our decision. On the way to the airport with tears in my eyes, I tried to call Brian ... again. His phone rolled to voicemail, and I wanted to scream. In times like this, I despise his job and the lack of availability that goes with it. I was sad and angry and disappointed, and not being able to reach him when I needed him most only added to my frustration. Despite the number of times I'd tried to reach him, he hadn't been able to answer all morning and wasn't even aware of Will's EEG results.

We arrived at the airport, and I was desperately trying to hold it together, not wanting to bring down our birthday crew. We'd been planning this trip for so long, and she was the first of our friends to enter our 40s. Then, Brian finally called me back and all bets were off. I couldn't stop the tears from falling once again. We went back and forth about the diet and drugs, but we couldn't reach an agreement. I was feeling stressed from the difficult day and was not in a good place to have a serious discussion. We cut the call short and ended on a pretty tough note. I felt bad about it later, but I needed to clear my head and get myself together. A couple of cocktails on the plane were definitely in order.

The weekend in Chicago was great. That town really reminds me of good times! I loved visiting Brian there when he played for the Chicago White Sox. It was such an amazing time in our lives, and I relished the opportunity to relive those feelings as I walked around that awesome city. I was relieved to learn that Will was doing fine at home. I couldn't help but check in a million times; I felt helpless being so far away. Brian ended up having to work a ton, so my mom had the boys for most of the weekend. She gave me a more detailed report than I probably would have gotten from my husband, which I appreciated and needed for my peace of mind. I missed all three of my boys and was so glad everything was OK.

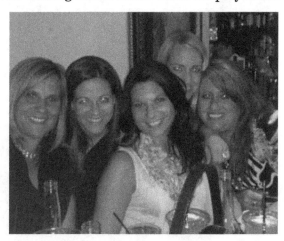

Girls' weekend in Chicago

Being with a great group of women helped to clear my mind. A day full of shopping on Michigan Avenue (retail therapy), deep dish pizza, and lots of laughs is exactly what I needed. Still, my mind was preoccupied with thoughts of home and the decisions that would have to be made on my return. I wished I could've been as happy-go-lucky as I usually am, but my friends were all understanding. I was scared of what was ahead of us, but I was also re-energized and ready to fight again. We'd figure this out and help get our sweet Will well. I kept reminding myself that tons of people have worse problems and to count the blessings we had. So, until next time Chi-town ... I love you!

# CHAPTER 18
# SCRATCH AND SNIFF

Will's relapse had caught us all by surprise. The file that we thought had been closed for good was suddenly reopened, and we were back at square one. After much debate, we decided to give the ketogenic diet another try. After all, the last time we initiated the keto diet, Will's seizures had ceased completely after only four days.

Still, Will was going to freak out when he learned of our decision. He'd been off the diet and thriving for almost a year, and now we were going to put him back on it—this time with full knowledge of how hard it truly was going to be. Will was seven years old now and more independent than ever. He would not want to give up the freedom to eat what he wanted, when he wanted, and without a fight.

With that in mind, Brian and I decided to tell Will of our decision one day and start the diet on the next. No point in delaying the inevitable and giving ourselves any excuse to change our minds. It'd be way too tempting to find an excuse not to do it. There was never going to be a good day to get started, but Brian and I looked at the calendar and chose July 3rd as *diet day*. Historically, July had always been a tricky month for Will for reasons that we couldn't fully understand or explain, but with his seizures getting worse, we didn't want to wait any longer to get started. Plus, Will was going to be surrounded by his biggest fans and cheerleaders over the long, holiday weekend—his family.

So, I dusted off my food scale and pulled my binder full of keto recipes out of the cupboard. It didn't take me long to get reacquainted with everything since I'd been offering advice to other families pursuing the ketogenic diet as a treatment for their own children. I'd been sharing the recipes and tips I learned along our journey and was now grateful to have maintained a level of familiarity. Will, on the other hand, had managed to block the entire experience out of his mind like a bad dream. You might well imagine Will's reaction when we finally broke the news—disbelief, disappointment, anger, and sadness.

But I had faith in this diet, despite the difficulties it presented, and I was confident the results would be worth the hardships. Or so I thought. Unfortunately, for no specific reason that anyone could determine, the ketogenic diet didn't work for Will this time. We followed it precisely for two full weeks, and even though he had achieved ketosis, Will's seizure count had increased. As a result, Brian and I agreed to stop the diet immediately and seek out another solution.

We met with his doctors that same week, and they agreed it was best to stop the diet. The stress of the whole situation was likely causing Will to seize more frequently, and that was unacceptable. We needed to do something to stem the tide of seizures that were wracking Will's brain and made the decision to start him back on Depakote, an anti-seizure drug that he tolerated in the past. We were back to the drawing board, and we were all nervous ... everyone except Will. He was thrilled to be off the ketogenic diet again.

The next couple of months were spent doctoring and researching. At one point, we were sent to a dermatologist because of a splotch of white pigmentation that'd been discovered on Will's back. That appointment didn't go so well. The dermatologist said that he was concerned Will might have Tuberous Sclerosis. Seriously? How could something so seemingly innocuous point to such a rare, multisystem genetic disease? The doctor recommended that we see a neurologist as soon as possible. I thought it had to be some sort of joke considering Will had been seeing a neurologist every month for the past two years. So, instead of blindly heading back to Children's Hospital, I called Will's nurse practitioner. She immediately put my mind at ease, informing me that they'd already crossed tuberous sclerosis off the list for Will some time ago during the numerous tests they'd conducted. *Thank God.* I'm not sure my heart could've taken the pain of discovering another serious ailment.

With a sigh of relief, we tried to piece together a somewhat normal existence. Will was happily eating to his heart's content, but his seizures continued to worsen. I dialed his doctor once again, desperately looking for answers. Sadly, they had none to offer. The only thing they could think of trying was an increase in the dosage of Will's medication. Brian and I were reluctant to do it but also at a loss as to what else we might try. Resigned, we upped Will's intake and prayed it would be the key to stopping his seizures. Within two days of the increase, Will started having accidents. Yes, at seven years old, our son was experiencing urinary incontinence, and he was mortified. He had no clue it was going to happen until it was too late. I was so nervous that it'd happen to him at school where the embarrassment and ruthless teasing would follow him forever. I went to the grocery store and picked up a pack of Depend® underwear. It felt so surreal as I stood in the check-out line buying adult diapers for my second grader. I wanted to protect him, but I guess I should've known he wouldn't even want to try them. What seven-year-old would want to be back in diapers?

Will was so upset about it we decided to keep him home from school for a day or two until we could figure something out. That first day home, he had six accidents; the following day he had seven. It had to be the meds, we deduced, and made the decision to immediately decrease the dosage again. His daily seizure count did decrease but at what cost? Unwelcome side effects were the main reason we wanted to get away from all medications from the start. Thankfully, within two days, the urinary incontinence stopped. Hallelujah! We were all so happy that Will had regained his bladder control that the fact that he was still seizing had seemed insignificant. It wasn't, of course, but at least now we were back to dealing with something we were familiar with and that most other people—at least those not trained to recognize absence seizures—might not even notice. For the next couple of months, we played with Will's doses and finally managed to get him to a good place. His seizures began to decrease in frequency and duration, and for that we were utterly thankful. Life was good, and we all tried our best to bask in the glow of blissfully uneventful days.

Then one day I got a call from Will's school nurse, Miss Mary. We'd been enjoying a couple months completely seizure free and I prayed that her call wasn't going to end that streak. Every time her number appeared on the caller id, I felt like I suffered a mild heart attack, and this time it was no different.

Miss Mary said, "Will is OK. He is just acting strange so I thought it would be best to let you know." She continued to explain the purpose of her call. Apparently, Will had smelled something terrible and claimed it'd made his mouth feel "funny." Being the great nurse that she is, Miss Mary knew that strange smells can be a part of a pre-seizure aura, known as an olfactory hallucination. Some people experience visual and hearing changes as well as numbness, anxiety, and nausea. Will had mentioned both visual and auditory changes in the past but never strange smells. I have learned over the years to never count anything out because his little brain is always evolving. Each seizure can be different than the next. Was this a warning sign of a seizure to come? I didn't know what to do. I had to assume that Will was going to start having seizures again and that those seizures might be foreshadowed by strange smells.

In the event my assumptions were right, I felt compelled to pop into school to check on Will when it was time to drop Blake off at the building for afternoon kindergarten. I snuck around the corner and said hello to the nurse, thanked her for the call, and asked how Will had been faring since then. She said he seemed to be doing fine and that she hadn't heard a thing since she'd sent him back to class.

The amazing school secretary overheard our conversation and offered to grab Will from the lunchroom for me so I could see for myself.

Will came skipping into the office as happy as could be and I was thrilled to see his smiling face. "Hi Mom!" he said. "What's up?" I proceeded to ask if he was OK, and he answered, "Why wouldn't I be?" When I reminded him that he'd spent some time with the nurse earlier that morning, he casually replied, "Oh, that was awful. I was reading this disgusting scratch and sniff book that had a picture of dirty socks in it. They smelled so gross, I almost puked!" I burst out with laughter, overcome with a rush of relief—no olfactory hallucination, no seizure—just smelly scratch-and-sniff socks and a crazy, hypochondriac mother. I had conditioned myself to continually brace for the worst, and I couldn't have been happier to find that day, I didn't have to.

If you've made it this far into our story, then I'm sure you've been feeling the ups and downs along with us. For every peak, there seems to be a valley: an endless cycle of setbacks that followed any progress. Sure enough, after reveling in the peace of several seizure-free months, they inevitably returned, and I had to ask myself, *would Will ever be free?*

At least this time I felt like I could attribute them to something more concrete and likely self-induced, like lack of sleep, which is a big trigger for Will. He had been having trouble falling asleep of late because, apparently, he'd been newly introduced to an old ghost story that was being spread around on the school bus and in the cafeteria—the legend of Bloody Mary. After two nights of Will pacing the halls, he came into our room and explained the problem: he was scared. He'd taken his friend's dare to look in a mirror and say, "Bloody Mary" three times in a row—an ineffectual conjuring of a nonexistent spirit. *Still*, it'd left him restless and unsettled: two things he couldn't afford to be when his brain and body needed that time to recover. I removed the mirror from his bedroom wall and tried to assure him that it was all just a silly myth. I even took him into the bathroom with me and said the words myself to prove it wasn't true.

Bloody Mary never answered our summons, but just be sure, we left the large light on in the hallway overnight to keep the spirits at bay. Will played his Mozart CD to help him fall asleep, and I would sleep with him on occasion. I was willing to do just about anything to get this kid a good night's sleep, even if it meant I didn't. Every night he'd pray to God to keep the nightmares away and to please heal his brain. I'd pray for the same—and so much more—trusting that God would answer ... someday.

# CHAPTER 19
# DIVINE INTERVENTION

*"The doctor of the future will give no medication but will interest his patients in the care of the human frame, diet and in the cause and prevention of disease."* [5]

*- Thomas Edison*

During this whole medical debacle, I often asked God to send me a sign so I would know which way to turn. When I wasn't *seeing* these signs or symbols, I felt desperate. I found myself grasping for straws or imagining indicators for the assurance I needed to make peace with the decisions we already made ... and the choices we still had to make. I'd be lying if I said that the stress didn't take a mental and physical toll on me.

I'd been prone to nasty headaches in the past, but now the throbbing in my head and pain in my neck had become unbearable. I needed to get some help and I knew just where to turn to get it. Thank God I had a great contact at my primary care doctor's office—my mom. Nonny was a nurse for the same practice at the time, and she helped me book an appointment immediately. In a matter of hours, I was meeting with a nurse practitioner who also happened to be a dear friend of my mom's.

The nurse practitioner was intimately aware of what was going on in our home and I knew she understood how important it was for me to take care of myself so I could take care of my family. After

---

[5] Thomas A. Edison, quoted in U.S. Medicine.
https://www.usmedicine.com/editor-in-chief/the-doctor-of-the-future-will-give/

going over my history of migraines, she suggested some possible solutions. After all the drugs we'd tried with Will, and the horrible side effects we witnessed, she knew that drugs wouldn't be an option for me. So, she suggested I consider other, less traditional forms of treatment. Specifically, she recommended massage therapy and chiropractic treatment. When my doctor ordered regular massages, how could I disobey? I was all about massages but a chiropractor? I had always wondered if a chiropractor could really help me but being married to Brian, whose job is dependent on conventional medicine, made it a tough sell. But as I sat in that office with yet another pounding headache, I decided I was going to do everything in my power to make him a believer. I was going to a masseuse and a chiropractor!

And then the sign I'd been so desperately searching for suddenly appeared. The chiropractor I had been referred to was someone I already knew. The nurse practitioner described the chiropractor as gentle and very knowledgeable, and she thought the two of us would click. It turns out that I grew up taking dance lessons from the doctor's mother! Once again, Pittsburgh proved to be one big, happy family. Feeling more comfortable and confident pursuing this option, I knew the only other thing I needed to do was to get Brian on board. We make medical decisions together and although this time it was about me, not Will, I still wanted his opinion and his blessing.

Surprisingly, it didn't take too much convincing. Brian agreed that I needed some relief from my headaches, and he was willing to see what she had to say. I didn't waste another moment before scheduling the appointment. I was anxious to get started and praying she could help me. It was strange to be going to a doctor to seek relief for my own ailments. The doctor was so welcoming and sweet, and she put me at ease almost immediately. I could tell that she understood what I was experiencing and was confident that she'd be able to help. After we discussed my issues and goals, she connected me to a diagnostic surface scanning electromyography

(EMG) machine and explained that the data it collected would show exactly what was going on with my head, neck, and back.

The test revealed that I indeed needed her help. I was all out of whack, and she was ready to go to work. She also believes in helping the whole person not just the specific complaint. During my chiropractic appointments, she'd always ask me what was going on in my life. It was already obvious to her that I'd been holding all my stress in my neck and back, but she wanted to dig deeper to understand the cause.

As I began to tell Will's story and share my fears, a lot of tears came pouring out. Embarrassed, I said, "I know you aren't that kind of doctor, but I guess it's safe to say I needed to talk to someone!"

She was so kind and calming. She really takes an interest in her patients' overall well-being rather than just focusing on their tissues and bones. She wanted to help, and I believed that she could. I felt like it was meant to be. I was ready to be healed—physically, mentally, and emotionally—and I knew in my heart that she'd be able to help make that happen.

I was avidly interested in learning about the complex relationship between the mind, body, and environment, and about how they worked together or against one another. With her help, I began to understand how my body needed to be reset, what I needed to do to give it some time to heal and adopt a new *normal*. It was so refreshing to speak with a medical professional who had an interest in holistic healing. She wanted more than to treat the symptoms of a problem, she wanted to cure the cause. Over the years, I'd become overwhelmed with Will's treatment options, so many of which had only managed to mask the pain. He deserved to feel well, preferably without drugs and their awful, unpredictable side effects. That's when I realized what we needed to do next for sweet Will—a consultation with my chiropractor!

She was cognizant of Brian's issues and concerns regarding the field of chiropractic care. She and I both knew it would be a challenge to get Brian's approval for her to treat Will. She offered to evaluate Will and provide a preliminary treatment plan, including a detailed diagram of Will's back and her explanation of what she thought might be going on in the hopes that it would help Brian to make an informed decision and give her a chance. She was right! Despite his skepticism and reservations, my trust in her was evident and unwavering. So, after a couple weeks of ongoing debate (i.e., me nagging), Brian chose to trust my instincts and consented.

I'm a big believer that there are certain people in the world that I'm supposed to know; that our paths were meant to cross and our lives to intertwine. Call it kismet—or providence—either way, the number of people that have come into my adult life and made a marked difference in it is too great to think that it wasn't preordained. I know without a doubt that this amazing, gentle chiropractor is one of those people for us. I prayed for a sign, for another option for Will, and she came into my life.

In my heart, I knew that drugs were not going to be the answer for Will. We'd changed his life already once before through diet alone. Though it was strict and exact, it was 100% natural. Just like this new treatment plan. Since I was a child, I'd always been a bit of a naturalist. Do I dye my hair? Yes. Do I have solar panels on my roof? No. But, I do believe the earth is full of wonders and remedies that most of us are either quick to dismiss or are simply unaware of. So, it was time to take a chance on another doctor; time to detox and reset Will's nervous system; time for Will to meet the chiropractor!

Will was apprehensive to see yet another doctor. I promised him (something I hated doing) that he would have a good experience. I knew she would make him feel comfortable and hopefully better all around. His first appointment was very similar to mine. She was gentle and informative and collected a large amount of data for his file—Will tends to have large files! Anyway, she also provided us with literature to look over at home and to show Brian.

She found a couple areas of concern, which were not surprising, and actually, her concern gave me hope—hope that she could actually provide some relief or calm his system. We took in everything that day and headed home to share the new chiropractic game-plan with Brian. Will was just relieved that he didn't have to get any shots or give any blood samples. It was an enjoyable appointment for him, and I was so grateful.

Brian concurred and we began treatment a few days later. We continued to see the chiropractor on a regular basis. We never could definitively say what was helping Will because we were trying so many treatments. However, I was confident that the chiropractor was on the doctor's good list. She was helping us both, and at this point, any help we could get was welcomed!

# CHAPTER 20
# IN THE SHADOWS

Having a child with an unpredictable and ongoing medical condition takes a toll beyond the child caught in the throes of the illness. There's a certain amount of collateral damage that affects nearly every family member including the parents, immediate caretakers, and siblings who inadvertently grow up in the shadows of an ailing brother or sister. I can say with certainty that Will never wanted to be the center of attention. My shy, quiet son had been forced into our family spotlight by the *bad guys* in his brain. Meanwhile, his younger brother Blake—who was still in my belly when Will had his first seizure—was just along for the ride. Even my pregnancy with Blake had been overshadowed with worry and concern for my first-born and fear that the second might suffer in a similar way.

Thank God, Blake was born healthy and remains so to this day. He's a sweet, funny, adorable, and energetic boy who'd been so patient through countless doctor's appointments, emotional breakdowns, and missed opportunities. He'd been a trooper through it all, and I'm so lucky and thankful for that. At the same time, it's been one of my biggest sources of guilt as a parent. We needed to do a better job of making Blake feel special. He would often say, "What about me?" and it broke my heart. All he wanted was a little of our time and attention, and he deserved that and so much more.

Even when we weren't in the midst of a medical crisis, we were always on the hunt for answers and debating treatment options for Will. The neurology department had recently recommended we put Will on a gluten-free diet to see if that might help. If it could make a difference, I was all for it! When I mentioned it to Will's long-term pediatrician, she suggested getting some blood work done first to gauge Will's tolerance to gluten while we did our own research.

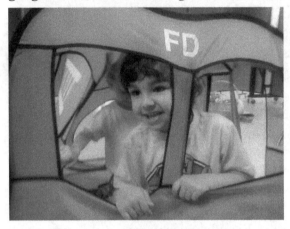

Our sweet Blake

Even though gluten-free diets aren't anywhere near as restrictive as a ketogenic diet, we weren't too keen on altering that aspect of his life without some evidence that it wouldn't cause more harm than good.

So, first thing the next morning we piled in the car and headed to the blood lab. Will's blood work required fasting levels, and I didn't want to make him suffer too long before he could have something to eat. Brian had already left for work so, once again, Blake had no choice but to go along for the ride.

When we got in the car, to my surprise, Will said, "I'm kind of excited to get blood work done."

Blake then asked, "Is it fun?"

I chuckled to myself as I listened to their crazy conversation. It's not exactly the kind of thing you'd expect two kids, ages five and eight, to animatedly discuss. Will claimed he never really minded it and that the nurses were usually very nice. Although he hadn't been talking to me, I was relieved all the same to know that the countless needle pricks he'd endured over the years hadn't pained him as much as I had imagined. When we arrived at the lab, Will offered his arm, and proceeded to fill four vials without so much as batting an eye. When he was done, I congratulated Will and gave him a hug.

Blake turned to me and asked, "What about me? Aren't you proud of me?"

I hugged him too and replied, "Of course we are, honey. Always."

And we truly were. He'd always been more patient and understanding than I ever imagined a kid his age could be. He'd always been a bit of a momma's boy and had a hard time understanding why I was the one who always had to stay with Will in the hospital overnight. Still, he loved spending time with his grandparents and cousins and stayed with them without complaint. Brian made sure to spend extra time with Blake. They were always outside playing catch or riding bikes together. They enjoyed their one-on-one time and made sure it happened often.

A few days later, Will's bloodwork came back and revealed that he had a sensitivity to wheat, milk, and eggs but no actual allergies. Still, we decided to give the gluten-free diet a try and hoped that it would work for Will. As you might imagine, he wasn't thrilled with going on any kind of restrictive diet again, and we weren't totally on board with depriving him just for the sake of it, so we opted to proceed with caution. For an eight-year-old, he was incredibly in tune with his body, and we were counting on that. We didn't want to make matters worse or cause him any undue stress. So, I did some research, drafted a shopping list, and headed to the store.

As I put Will to bed that night, he made sure to remind me that he'd hated the gluten-free pizza I'd made for dinner that night. I couldn't help but chuckle at that because, yeah, it wasn't a Chicago-style deep dish. He smiled back and said with all the certainty in the world, "But it's OK Mom. I'll only need to worry about it for five more months!" To my look of surprise, he explained that his seizures come and go but they'd definitely be gone by then. He's so great and optimistic. I could only hope and pray that he was right.

Given our unfortunate history, I shouldn't have been surprised at all when Will had the worst seizure we'd seen in a long time later that week. We were at Will's basketball game, and he was clearly struggling. His face was red, he was out of breath, and he appeared to be a bit off kilter. I wasn't sure if he was getting sick or if something more nefarious was going on. At one point, in the middle of the game, he started to walk directly toward the opposing team's

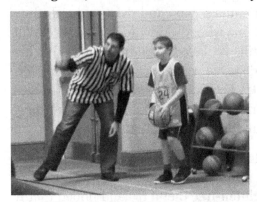

bench. His coach looked concerned and waved me over to investigate. I moved closer to the court to get a better look and was scared by what I saw. Will appeared to be noticeably dazed, his eyes were vacant and unfocused. A moment later, he stumbled to the ground and when he got up, he started to cry. I rushed

"Will the Thrill" and his referee dad

onto the court and ushered him out of the gym. Thankfully Brian's parents were with us, so Blake stayed with them and continued to watch the game. I sat Will on the floor in the hallway and prepped him just in case a seizure was coming. Once he calmed down and caught his breath he said, "Something is wrong, Mommy. My brain isn't sending signals to my body, and it's really scary."

We think he experienced a seizure, and it was the first time he'd actually been aware of it happening. He'd never recalled any of the countless seizures he'd had in the past, and we were both a bit shocked by this new revelation. Whatever was going on in his brain had freaked him out and left him feeling unsettled and disoriented. I felt the same way to be perfectly honest. After a ten-minute rest, Will had collected himself and was ready to head back into the gym.

He was not, however, ready to get back into the game. Instead, Will asked the coach if he could be the score keeper. He did a great job from the bench, and I did everything I could to hold back my tears.

The following week, Brian and I were scheduled to travel to Arizona for my cousin's wedding. Once again, we were faced with the decision of whether we should stay or go. The arrangements had been made weeks ago for the boys to stay with Grandma and G-Daddy during our three-day trip, but with Will's latest seizure fresh on our minds, we were hesitant to be so far away. At the end of the day, Brian and I knew that both kids would be in good hands at *Camp Grandparents* and decided that a little getaway and some southwestern sunshine could do a world of good for us both.

So, we packed up all of Will's meds and supplements while the boys packed a mountain of blankets and stuffed animals. Because I had already purchased all the ingredients, I decided to make up some gluten-free meals for Brian's parents to serve to Will in our absence. I wasn't surprised to learn that Will would rather enjoy grandma's delicious cooking and forgo the less-than-desirable, gluten-free foods that I'd left behind for him. I was surprised, however, by the endless stream of voice calls, video chats, and text messages I received from Will after touching down in Arizona to reiterate his displeasure. Brian and I decided then and there that we didn't want to cause Will any added stress while we were away, so, as we hiked through the rock formations on the first morning of our trip, we told Will that he could drop the diet and eat whatever he wanted. He was ecstatic and we were relieved—hopeful that everyone could fully enjoy the next couple of days without worry.

When my phone rang again only a few minutes later, I sighed deeply with exasperation—certain that it was Will calling yet again—until I saw that it was actually my mom on the line. She sounded upset as she asked where Brian and I were. I told her that we were on our way back from our morning hike but were still at least three miles away. Once she realized we weren't at the hotel, she tried to avoid telling me the reason why she'd called, but hearing the shaky strain in her voice, I knew that something was wrong.

"What's going on? Is everyone ok?" I asked.

That's when she told me that my dad was on his way to the hospital. He and my brother had decided to visit my brother's best friend, who happened to live in Scottsdale where we were all staying for the wedding. My brother explained that my dad had started acting strange shortly after they'd arrived at his house. He asked for a glass of water and fainted before he had a chance to drink it. They immediately called 911 and

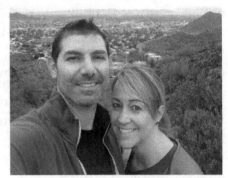

A moment of peace

within minutes an ambulance, fire truck, and police officer arrived to tend to my dad and get him to the emergency room. Since we only had one car to transport all of us, my brother had to rush back to the hotel to pick up my mom, sister, and her husband while his friend rode in the ambulance with my dad to the hospital. Luckily, he is a surgeon at the hospital and was able to make sure that my dad was taken in for treatment right away.

In the meantime, Brian and I made our way back down the mountain path as fast as we could safely go. It didn't feel real. We'd gone to Arizona to escape hospitals and doctors for a few days and here we were racing to the ER for my dad. I was filled with worry and emotion and couldn't get there to see him soon enough. We made it off the trail just in time to hop in the car with the rest of my family. When we arrived at the hospital, I was flooded with relief to learn that my dad was OK. That said, the source of his distress was still unclear. The doctors did some tests and took blood samples to get to the bottom of it. It might've been a heart attack. As we waited for the results, the nurse set him up with an IV to rehydrate him.

After three hours, my dad was feeling well enough to be released from the ER. The doctors diagnosed him with a simple case of dehydration but urged him to follow up with a cardiologist in Pittsburgh. Shortly after we returned to our hotel, it was time for the wedding. Though none of us really felt like kicking up our heels, we'd traveled all that way to celebrate with our extended west coast family, and that's precisely what we were going to do.

We ended up having a great time despite my dad's dampened energy. He's usually the life of the party, so it was sad to see him sitting tiredly at a table instead of in the middle of a crowd regaling everyone with his stories. It was a wake-up call for me as it was the first time I realized and acknowledged that my parents aren't invincible. Aging is inevitable, as are ailments that attack our bodies and minds as time ticks by. Yet another reminder to live in the moment and be thankful for the good things in life. It's all so fragile and fleeting. With those thoughts fresh in my mind, we could hardly wait to head home and be back with our boys. Our getaway hadn't gone as planned, but that was par for the course.

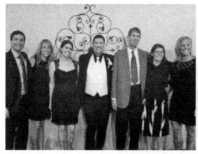 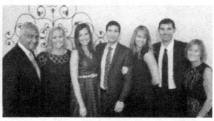

Cousins (left),     Family time (right)

# CHAPTER 21
# CAN YOU HEAR ME NOW?

Once we returned from Arizona, things calmed down for a while; however, life still moved fast, and our boys were growing up. My dad's health had stabilized, and Will's seemed to have as well. Both boys were excelling in school and enjoying their sports. We spent our evenings going between baseball diamonds and soccer fields and enjoying every hectic, healthy minute of it. When an assistant coach position opened on Blake's team, I jumped at the opportunity to finally be able to do something just for Blake. I loved watching him play, and I had a blast coaching his team of super-charged six-year-olds. The head coach, Jim, and I always joked that I was more of a team mom than a coach, but the title didn't matter to me. I was on the field every game, and it made both Blake and me incredibly happy.

I have no illusions that our contentment, both then and now, is mostly contingent on Will's good health. The days he was well, we were all happy; the days when he wasn't, neither were we. Truth be told, I hate how Will's ailments have the power to manipulate our moods—especially my own. I hate how wary I've become, always waiting for the proverbial floor to fall out from under our feet. Even on good days, I find myself searching for signs of the next catastrophe.

Will sensed my enduring apprehension and didn't want to make matters worse, at least that's why I think he decided not to tell me the next time he didn't feel well.

One day he finally came to me and admitted, "Mom, I didn't want to have to worry you about this, but my ears have been really bothering me for the last two months. I hate to see you upset about me, but I feel like I've been on an airplane and can't pop my ears."

Two months! I was simultaneously touched by his concern for my nerves and appalled that he'd been so worried about them and suffered in silence for so long. Especially with something that I assumed could be easily remedied with a course of antibiotics.

Will had been swimming at an indoor pool during a recent getaway, and his symptoms pointed to swimmer's ear or possibly an ear infection. Even though he'd said it had been bothering him for a couple of months, I decided to wait a couple more days to see if it would miraculously go away on its own. A girl can always dream right? Unfortunately, his pain continued, and he seemed to be feeling worse. Not wanting Will to suffer another minute, I called the pediatrician to get the diagnosis ball rolling. I wasn't sure if I should feel relieved or worried when his doctor couldn't see much wrong. His ears didn't appear to be infected but every time she touched them, Will winced in pain. She noticed that his left sinus cavities were congested and thought that could be contributing to the pressure he'd been feeling. She suggested that we try a prescription nasal spray to alleviate the pressure in his sinuses. Will wasn't particularly excited about using nasal spray, but after weeks of pain, he was willing to try anything.

He used the spray faithfully for a full week, but nothing had changed. He was still trying to pop his ears and still experiencing pain and headaches. He was uncomfortable but felt well enough to muscle through each school day. When I called the pediatrician back, the nurse recommended regular doses of Motrin to help him manage the pain, so that's what we did. We still didn't know what had been causing the pain, but at least we were doing our best to treat it. He seemed to be getting by, and then I got a call from the school nurse.

I happened to be at the school for a PTA meeting that morning and had just made my way out to my car. I checked my phone and noticed that I had a missed a call from the nurse, so I turned on my heel and headed back inside. I found Will laying on the couch in the nurse's office with a heating pad on his face. Poor guy! Miss Mary, the nurse, said he had been lying there for a half hour in pain. When I didn't answer my phone the first time, Will said he thought I might be at Sam's Club because I don't get much service inside of the store. In hindsight, it's kind of funny that he'd make that assumption because I do spend a lot of time shopping at Sam's. Still, at the time I felt terrible. He needed me, and I was just down the hall. At least I hadn't left the parking lot yet!

I took Will home with me and resumed the search for answers. I called the pediatrician again to let her know that the nasal spray wasn't helping as we'd hoped. With the thought that Will might be suffering from a possible infection, she decided to prescribe him an antibiotic. So, off to the pharmacy I went once again. Will was thrilled to be rid of the nasal spray and had become so practiced at taking *horse pills* that he wasn't put off in the slightest at having to take a few more now, especially if they'd take his pain away.

After becoming familiar with Will and his luck—or lack thereof—with quick fixes, I'm sure you won't be surprised to learn that after a week on the antibiotics, his symptoms had actually gotten worse. The pain had become so bad, I opted to keep him home from school. Another, more desperate call to the pediatrician ended with me scheduling an appointment at Children's Hospital with an ear, nose, and throat (ENT) specialist. Surely, they'll know what's going on with Will, right?

Wrong. We spent roughly three hours at the ENT, during which time Will underwent an exam, a hearing test, and an ear pressure test. With the results in hand, the ENT claimed everything looked perfect. I could hardly concentrate as he spoke, my mind was whirling with panic. I began to question my sanity. Was I going crazy? I peered suspiciously at Will's medical file and wondered if there was a sticky note inside somewhere that read, *Beware: delusional mother.* Did this ENT doctor think I was making this up, or worse that Will was faking his symptoms in some ploy for attention? How, after months of unidentified pain, could Will appear to be the picture of health? Seizures excluded, of course. It was all so strange yet so perfectly par for the course with our son. I blinked back to attention after the doctor had delivered what should have been good news and asked, "So, where do we go from here?"

The doctor went on to explain that since the source of his pain was not connected to his ears, there was a good possibility that it could be connected to the joint *next* to the ear. It was his opinion that Will might be suffering from temporomandibular joint (TMJ) pain. With that, he signed off on Will's file and recommended that we follow up with a dentist or orthodontist. Will looked confused and deflated as we gathered our things and left the office.

When we got to the car, he turned to me and said, "Why am I always so hard to figure out? What's wrong with me?"

I hated hearing those questions from his sweet little mouth, but I must admit that I'd been wondering the exact same thing.

I pasted on my best, reassuring smile and replied, "I don't know, sweetie, but we'll figure it out."

By that time, it was nearly noon, so rather than rushing Will back to school, I decided to take him to lunch and let him have the rest of the day off. Will was happy to rent a movie and head home for a little rest and relaxation, and I just needed a moment to unwind. I was still stunned by the news that his ears were just fine and determined to learn what I could about TMJ. Even though I know better than to seek specific answers to vague medical questions online, I found it impossible to avoid the temptation. So, I booted up my laptop and began to click around, harvesting WebMD and other medical websites for signs and symptoms of TMJ.

It didn't take long to learn that sure enough, ear fullness and pain are key indicators of TMJ. Turns out, many of the symptoms associated with TMJ lined up with what Will had been experiencing. I could feel a sense of relief wash over me as the puzzle pieces began to fall into place. That was tempered with the knowledge that Will was still in pain. As we cuddled up together to watch the movie with our gas log fireplace pouring warmth into the room, I decided to call the dentist. The dentist asked if we could come in right away so she could rule out the possibility of an infection. Outside of ruining our quiet afternoon on the couch, we had no other excuse not to go then. We shut everything down in the house and hopped in the car to head to another appointment. As we pulled out of the driveway, my thoughts shifted to Blake and the fact that he'd be getting off the bus in a couple of hours. I hoped we'd be back in time to greet him, but I placed a call to our amazing neighbors to be ready just in case. Again, the guilt of treating our second child as an afterthought ate away at my conscience. I took solace in the fact that he'd be in good hands and was the kind of kid that wouldn't be upset at me for arranging an impromptu playdate until we could pick him up.

Will and I were both relieved that he didn't have to wait long before the dentist took him back and got a good look in his mouth. When she pushed her chair back and pulled down her mask, she explained that he had a lot going on behind his lips. Loose teeth, moving teeth, incoming molars and not much space for them to grow into. She also said that the joint connecting his jaw felt like it was inflamed and agreed that the likely culprit causing Will's pain was, in fact, a case of TMJ. We left the office with a treatment plan that included Motrin, a mouth guard, and a referral to a local orthodontist. I was feeling vindicated (I wasn't going crazy!), but Will was just plain sad. "Another type of doctor?" he asked, as we clicked in our seatbelts for the short ride home. He'd been such a trooper throughout the entire, trying day. He'd been poked and prodded and passed from one doctor to the next. I couldn't blame the kid for feeling exasperated. Luckily, we were able to beat the bus home and waited for Blake by the curb. Blake was surprised to see his brother waiting for him and wondered why Will wasn't in school. Will bounced on the balls of his feet pleased as punch and bragged, "Mom let me skip!"

Blake, not surprisingly, was hurt and upset—angry at the injustice of not being allowed to skip school as well. I reminded him that Will had a doctor's appointment and that he hadn't been feeling well. Seemingly satisfied, Blake quickly moved on, dropping his backpack to pick up his basketball. Thank God he is so resilient.

As Will collapsed on the couch to resume his abandoned movie, I reviewed the list of treatment options his dentist provided to see which ones, if any, I could try to implement now to give him some relief. The first one was easy: provide Will with a mouth guard to prevent him from grinding his teeth in his sleep. Given the number of sports our boys both play, I'd bought each of them a mouth guard before the start of their last baseball season which neither of them ended up using. So, I dug around Will's baseball bag and found his mouth guard. As I suspected, it was still in its original packaging. I gave the first-use directions a quick glance as I listened to voicemail and grabbed Will some Motrin. It seemed simple enough—boil some water and drop the mouth guard in. Apparently, I'd missed a crucial piece of information as I attempted to multitask. No more than five minutes after I'd dropped the mouth guard into the pot on the stove then the house filled with the sickening smell of burnt rubber. I raced to the kitchen to find an unrecognizable ball of rubber roiling around in the pot. I took the pot off the burner and grabbed the empty mouth guard package out of the trash can to reread the instructions. I was supposed to put it in the water for 30 to 60 seconds, not five minutes! Good thing the hockey store is only a five-minute drive from the house. At least I'll know what not to do next time I go to sterilize it!

After I dumped the disgusting rubber mess down the drain and cracked open a couple of windows, I grabbed my phone to make a couple of calls. I reached out to a few friends who use orthodontists hoping that one of them would be able to take Will on as a new patient sooner rather than later. The first one I called said that they referred TMJ patients to someone outside of their practice ... figures! Since I'm fairly certain that Will is going to need braces someday, I wanted to get him established with an orthodontist that could see him through both issues. Then I remembered that one of my college roommates was married to an orthodontist in Raleigh. Brian suggested I give him a call. This guy loves teeth and talking about them, and he was more than happy to provide some recommendations. He was even acquainted with a doctor who could treat Will and would be willing to share notes with him so he could follow Will's case. I couldn't think of a better choice! It felt good to finally have a plan in place. Now all I had to do was keep Will comfortable until it was time for his appointment: no hard or chewy food, alternate between ice and heat treatments as needed, Motrin to help manage the pain, and a mouth guard when he sleeps.

I really hoped the mouth guard would help. On those nights when I used to sleep in Will's room—the nights I worried he might have a grand mal seizure—I used to listen helplessly as Will ground his teeth. The spine-tingling sound of crunching and squeaking would often wake me up out of a sound sleep. I'd try to wake Will up to get him to stop but it never worked. It was impossible to tell if the grinding was spurred by his seizure disorder or the medications he was on; maybe it was neither. Will has so many mysteries that we just can't seem to solve, but one thing is for sure, we'll never stop trying!

# Chapter 22
## Locker Debacle

In the weeks that followed Will's harrowing day playing hooky from school, things started to settle down. His seizures subsided and the pain he'd been experiencing in his ear and jaw had diminished. We made a few small, easy changes, and they seemed to help. We eliminated chewing gum, avoided super chewy snacks and foods, and gave him anti-inflammatory meds as needed for pain. It seemed like he experienced the worst pain after swimming, so I made it my mission to keep his ears healthy and dry all summer.

We'd managed to minimize Will's pain to the point that it was more of a minor inconvenience, and he seemed to be enjoying his summer. In fact, for the first time in a long while, we all were. Summers had always been difficult in the past, with Will suffering the worst of his seizures in the heat and humidity. As such, the pool simply wasn't an option, but with his epilepsy ostensibly under control, we did our best to make up for lost time. The boys and I created a summertime bucket list, filled with activities we'd intentionally avoided in the past and tried to complete it while everyone was healthy.

We spent many days at the pool and most of our evenings at the ballpark. Will and Blake were both playing baseball, and I relished the chance to watch them have fun with their friends on warm summer nights. Even so, I couldn't help but be a bit nervous every time Will took to the field. Especially, the few times when a ball was headed straight for his face, and he didn't seem to be aware it was coming. On the days he was first baseman, I felt compelled to sit by the first-base line to shout a warning to Will when the ball was hit toward him.

Even though we didn't want to admit it, it was evident his absence seizures had returned, and Will sometimes had them on the field. Will's coach was awesome. He was very observant and as soon as he noticed Will staring off into space, he'd alert me immediately or stop play until Will had a chance to get himself together. I vividly remember one night when Will had been pitching and had two small seizures on the mound. I knew from experience that the staring spells would pass, and that Will would take them in stride. So, when his coach called out, "Mom! Will's mom!" I held up my hand to acknowledge that I'd heard him and kept my eyes fixed on my son. His coach and I exchanged glances as we waited to see how Will would respond. Luckily, I was right, and Will did exactly what I thought—he blinked his eyes, repositioned himself on the mound, and wound up to throw the next pitch. He was not about to let his seizures ruin his game or control his life!

As the pitch sailed toward home plate, I didn't know whether I wanted to cheer or cry. I'm sure that no one else watching the game even knew that he'd been seizing and for that I was so thankful. With the support and empathy of Will's coach, he'd made it through the season without any injuries or traumatic episodes despite the unpredictable nature of his condition. Thinking back, we'd been blessed with so many great coaches over the years; each one played an important role in teaching our sons about good sportsmanship and the importance and value of teamwork. This particular year was no exception, and, with the help of their coaches, both Will and Blake had decent seasons. Brian and I were so proud of their hard work—during and between games—especially Blake's. He always jumped at the opportunity to go with his dad to practice. Not only did they hone their skills, but it helped to pass the time on the long, waning days of summer.

Soon enough, summer was over, and the new school year was about to begin. While Blake was bummed that their long vacation was ending, Will was super excited to start fifth grade in the bigger, air-conditioned intermediate school. I wasn't all that surprised considering Will's zeal for learning and Blake's enthusiasm for recess. During the first week, I made an appointment to meet with the intermediate school nurse to discuss Will's condition. She was knowledgeable, empathetic, and confident—everything I could hope for during Will's transition to a bigger building with a much larger student body.

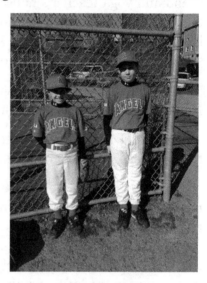

"The Angels"

After we'd discussed Will's history, I let her know about the handful of absence seizures he'd been experiencing every day for the past few weeks. Even though he seemed to be able to bring himself out of the usually brief episodes, the nurse suggested revisions to his seizure action plan that included keeping Will's emergency meds in her office. Will was thrilled to learn that he no longer needed the anal Diastat medication prescribed since he was a preschooler and had been terrified of needing for just as long. Due to his size he was prescribed an emergency nasal spray instead. Will wasn't alone in his sense of relief, I was ecstatic that he wouldn't be subjected to any added humiliation if he were to have a grand mal seizure, which would be mortifying enough. I'm sure the school nurse was relieved as well!

With an action plan in place, the school year began, and the first week went by in a blur. Will loved his new school and both boys settled in nicely. Everyone was happy, and then one day the following month, all our worst fears came true—Will had a grand mal seizure at school.

Over the years, I've received countless calls from school nurses but none of them were as frightening as this one. I had just left my friend and yoga teacher's house where I'd been acting as a subject for her Tai massage therapy hours (lucky me!) and headed home, happy and relaxed. Suddenly, I received an incoming call I could see was coming from Will's school.

I'd barely had a chance to say hello when Will's teacher blurted, "Mrs. Simmons, Will is having a seizure, could you get here ASAP?"

My heart froze in my chest as I gripped the steering wheel tightly. "Yes," I replied in an instant. "I'll be there as fast as I can."

I ended the call and stepped on the gas, grateful to only have been about two minutes away from the building. As I parked the car and jogged toward the building, I imagined Will appearing catatonic. Sometimes he had staring spells that came in clusters and would leave him worryingly unresponsive. I imagined I'd find him resting in the office, waiting for me to come and check on him. With that in mind, I was not at all prepared for the scene I was about to walk into.

As I walked hurriedly toward the entrance of the school, the front door swung open, and a teacher ran out to greet me.

She said, "Mrs. Simmons, right? Follow me!"

We bypassed the front office—something parents aren't normally allowed to do for security reasons—and headed straight for the hallway. As soon as we turned the corner, I saw Will laying on the floor in a full blown, convulsive, grand mal seizure. I couldn't believe my eyes. The wonderful school nurse was kneeling right next to him, as were two of his amazing teachers and an aid who happened to be an old neighbor of ours. I dropped to the ground and scooped Will up gently into my arms. My poor, sweet angel. As he began to blink back to consciousness, he looked so confused and utterly defeated. It shattered my heart into a million pieces. I checked him over for obvious injuries and, seeing none, refused the offer to call an ambulance. The seizure had ended, and I knew what to do.

What I *wanted* to do was whisk him away and remove him from the situation as fast as possible. He'd gone limp in my lap like a rag doll, drooling uncontrollably, as he faded in and out of awareness right there in the locker-lined hall. I did a quick check once he fully came to, to see if he'd lost control of his bladder as that tended to happen when he'd had grand mal seizures in the past. Thank God, for whatever reason, that had not happened this time. I wanted to sob with relief as I looked toward the heavens and said a silent prayer of thanks that he'd been spared that humiliation in front of his peers.

As the teachers and staff directed the students back toward their classrooms, the nurse retrieved a wheelchair and helped me to slowly get poor Will up off the floor. We wheeled him to the nurse's office to give him a little privacy and give me an opportunity to learn exactly what had happened. I wanted to know how long he'd been seizing before I arrived. Still feeling shaky, I called Brian to let him know what happened and make sure he agreed with my decision to forego the ambulance. As luck would have it, I couldn't get hold of him, so I hung up and called my parents instead. They answered immediately and were already getting into their car before we hung up the phone. I thought it would be best if someone sat in the back seat with Will to keep a watchful eye on him while I drove us either to the hospital or home. My next call was to his neurologist. Again, it rolled into voicemail. I was so frustrated I wanted to scream, *Please, someone answer. This is important!*

As soon as my parents pulled up to the school, the nurse and my mom helped me get Will into the car. I overheard the murmured whispers from the students walking through the halls as we led him toward the door. They were saying Will's name, and it put me on edge. I needed to get him out of there fast. Nonny hopped in the back seat with her grandson, and my dad followed us home. After I pulled the car into the garage, we helped Will into the house and onto the couch. He was still extremely groggy and appeared to still be experiencing some small seizures as well. He looked pallid and drained: completely exhausted by the battle his brain and body were waging without his consent. As soon as his head hit the pillow, he fell fast asleep. I knelt beside him for a moment and just stared at his face. He looked so peaceful resting safely here at home. Lord knows he needed it after the morning that he had. I kissed his forehead and willed his brain to rest and recover before stepping away to gather myself.

I chatted with my parents for a bit and thanked them again for their never-ending help and support. With a promise to keep them posted, I hugged them goodbye and went back to check on Will. He was still out cold, as expected. It wasn't unusual for him to sleep for an hour or more following a grand mal seizure. During his nap, I received a call back from his neurologist's office. They concurred with my decision that, unless something unexpected happened and Will took a turn for the worse, it wasn't necessary to make a trip to the ER. Still, they were anxious to see him as soon as possible, and I couldn't wait either. His seizures were getting worse and that was unacceptable. We needed to reevaluate his medication and treatment plan, and we needed to do it soon.

Shortly after I booked our appointment, the phone rang again. This time it was the school nurse. After we'd left the building, she went to work gathering as much information about what had happened as she could and had kindly called to relay what she'd learned.

Apparently, Will had been standing at his locker after lunch when the seizure began. The girl who had the locker next to his witnessed the whole thing and provided a very detailed account.

She said that she asked Will a question about their upcoming math class, and rather than reply, he just stood there and stared at her. She joked with him and said, "Hellllooooo, Will. Are you in there? What's for math?"

Then without saying a word, he clutched at his own stomach and fell to his knees. The next thing she knew, he was on the ground convulsing. Thankfully, his best friend Jack was just up the hall at his own locker when Will went down. Most of Will's classmates thought he was goofing around, but Jack knew better. He knew that Will needed help. Jack told everyone to step away from Will as he ran into the nearest classroom to get a teacher. The teacher acted fast, ordering everyone in the hallway to go into the closest classroom immediately to give Will a wide berth while he seized. Meanwhile, the nurse had been alerted and ran to the scene with Will's emergency meds in hand, and that's when I arrived to find my son seizing on the floor and drooling everywhere. It was a horrific sight; one I would be happy to never ever witness again. Since his seizure only lasted two to three minutes, his emergency meds did not need to be administered. They come into play after four minutes.

Will slept for two solid hours before he awoke, understandably confused as to why he was home on the couch instead of in school. Otherwise, he seemed rested and alert. I was so happy to see his eyes bright and open, not rolled back in his head. I laid with him on the couch for a moment to explain what had happened and answer any of his questions. He was embarrassed and upset, worried about what his classmates thought of him. Word of Will's seizure had indeed spread like wildfire, but instead of the teasing he expected, there was an outpouring of support. The school, the community, our neighbors, and our friends were all concerned for Will's health and wishing him well. Will's principal even called our home that evening to check on him. He shared his perspective on what had happened after Will left, telling him how the teachers had explained his disorder to his concerned classmates and did their best to answer questions. Will's friends were quick to squash the rumors and exaggerations that had spread in the aftermath—that Will had fallen down the stairs or fainted in the hall. We truly appreciated everything the staff and students did that day to help Will and set the record straight, especially his buddy Jack.

Though Will seemed to be feeling much better, I was terrified to put him to bed that night. I knew I'd never get a wink as I worried about him seizing in his sleep. So, I crawled under the covers with him in his room and kept watch as he slept. It took everything in me not to break down and cry, to scream at the world for the ways Will had suffered. Instead, I stared up at the ceiling and said a prayer. *Please let me take these seizures on myself. Don't let my son suffer anymore.*

As I laid there trying to hold myself together, I took comfort in the ongoing stream of text and Facebook messages that kept lighting up my phone in the dark of the night. It was so nice to read such kind words from so many caring people. They reminded me once again that we had a warrior in our midst. No matter how many times Will got knocked down, he always got up to fight another day … and we'd be right there with him.

# CHAPTER 23
# THE AFTERMATH

Brian and I decided to keep Will home for a couple days to recover. Physically, he was feeling alright, but I could tell that his ego had taken a bigger blow. Despite repeated assurances from his school principal, nurse, teachers, and his friends that it wasn't a big deal, Will still felt embarrassed and dreaded facing his classmates. I tried to convince him that everyone would be kind and that they'd be happy to see him back in the building healthy and happy and no worse for the wear. Unconvinced, yet unable to make a case to miss another day, Will returned to school before the end of the week.

Fortunately, I was correct for once! His teachers and classmates welcomed him back with open arms just as I'd hoped. His teacher sent me an email midmorning to let me know that he was having a great day. The other students all acted like nothing had happened, and I couldn't have been happier. I really appreciated that his teacher had taken time out of her hectic day to touch base and let me know how he was faring. It was nice to know that I'd find his smiling face that afternoon when he stepped off the bus.

We had a neurology appointment scheduled in a couple weeks and were all doing our best to just go about our lives. That included taking Will back to the ENT for his follow up visit. I was reminded once again of the pain and fullness that Will had said he still felt in his ears. The ENT suggested having tubes implanted to try and alleviate the pressure. At that point, I was willing to try anything if it would make Will feel better somehow and this seemed like a fairly easy fix. I'd apparently pushed Will's seizure troubles to the back of my mind when I scheduled surgery for him before leaving the office that day, not only to insert ear tubes but to remove his adenoids as well. I mean, why not kill two birds with one stone?

The next day, I was quickly reminded that the unpredictability of Will's epilepsy was something we couldn't simply schedule around. We needed to figure that out first and get it under better control before he went under the knife for even the most routine of surgeries. There was a much more serious problem here and we needed to focus.

I walked into our game room and found Will there, cleaning up a mess. Curious, I asked, "What's going on buddy?" He claimed that he had spilled his drink, but as I looked around the room, I could see no evidence that there had ever been a drink to clean up. I walked over to take a closer look and realized he'd had an accident and had been too embarrassed to tell me. Poor guy! I felt so bad for him. Though I didn't see it happen, it's safe to assume that Will had a seizure and lost control of his bladder in the process. I knew that Will was already upset and did my best not to make matters worse. So, I shrugged it off, cleaned up the mess, and tried to assure him that we'd sort everything out soon.

Of course, it never felt like soon enough and having to wait to see the neurologist wasn't helping any. I tried to beg for an earlier appointment but was not granted one. Unfortunately, we weren't considered a priority as there was a queue of kids deemed sicker than Will that needed to be seen first. I do understand that there are always others who are (sadly) in a worse way than Will. That knowledge did little to quell the frustration I felt as I could do nothing but watch my son's seizures return with a vengeance while we waited to be seen.

With each passing day, things seemed to only get worse. It got to the point that we didn't feel comfortable when Will was out of our sight. It didn't take much convincing to get him to agree to bring his Xbox from the game room we had built in the basement to the upstairs first-floor family room. He said, "I'm going to play one more round then I'll unplug it and can move it upstairs."

Satisfied with that plan, I nodded my approval and went back to making dinner. About ten minutes later, I heard a loud ruckus coming from the basement. I wasn't sure if it was just the sound of Will packing things up, so I grabbed a basket of clean laundry that needed to go upstairs and made my way to the third floor. I'd just made it to the top of the landing when I heard another bang, this one even louder than the first. The hairs on my arms stood on end as it dawned on me that something was wrong. I ran down the stairs and found Will stumbling through the foyer. As soon as I reached him, he collapsed in my arms and seized. I lowered him slowly to the floor and started counting as I learned to do. He came around within a minute and tried to talk to me, but his speech was slurred, and his words were jumbled. I rocked him in my arms and murmured words of encouragement until he had calmed down enough to safely move him to the couch in the family room. Maybe after the last couple of months I should've expected this to happen, but honestly, I felt as shocked as I was the day he'd had a grand mal seizure at school. How could this be happening again?

After Will resurfaced, I asked him if he remembered what had happened. He said that he'd been playing his game and got angry when he'd lost. That was the last thing he could recall. Once Brian got home from work and could sit with Will for a little, I ventured downstairs to check out the playroom. I was floored by what I saw. The room had been essentially wrecked. His gaming chair had been flipped over, the TV was left teetering on the edge of the entertainment center, and our sizable collection of remotes, controllers, cords, and headsets were haphazardly scattered all over the room. My poor child had felt his seizure coming on and had tried his damnedest to get to me for help. I couldn't stop the tears that rolled down my face as I stood in the center of the room turning slowly to survey the damage. The guilt that I felt nearly brought me to my knees as I imagined all the ways it could've been worse; the ways Will could've been hurt in the sanctity of his own home; and how frightened he must have been flailing and alone.

The sound of his voice echoing from the floor above me jolted me to action. I got to work, quickly cleaning up the mess before he'd have a chance to come downstairs and see it for himself. As I put things back in their proper places, I took a deep breath and decided then and there that I was going to call the neurologist, and I wasn't going to hang up until they agreed to see us as soon as possible.

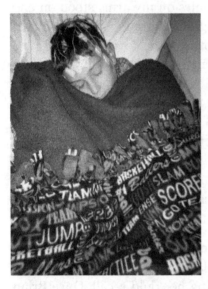

Catching some z's during an EEG

Fortunately, I didn't really need to plead my case. When the neurologist learned about the grand mal seizures Will had experienced, they wanted to see him right away. He was hooked up to the EEG again, and they witnessed his seizures. The very next day, we sat in their office and were relieved when they decided to put him back on Depakote. Even though we never wanted to medicate our son, fearful of unwanted side effects and wary of their effectiveness, now we felt we had no choice. We needed to do something to stop his seizures.

I couldn't get to the pharmacy fast enough to pick up his anti-seizure prescription. I know I've said it before, but our pharmacists are simply the best. After trying a wide variety of meds, they were keenly aware of which brands sat best with Will and worked to secure those particular pills for us every single time. It made me feel better knowing that they had our backs and would do what they could to make sure the medication didn't upset Will's stomach unnecessarily. When we got home and handed Will his first dose, I said a silent prayer. *Please Lord, let this work.* We'd conquered this beast a couple of times already and knew we could do it once more. Hopefully, for good this time.

A week on the medication and Will's seizures had started to decrease. I was so happy and grateful for the obvious improvement. Still, we'd been around the block enough times to know that it was too early to determine whether the effects would stay steady and keep his epilepsy at bay. Following Will's grand mal seizure in school, the administrators suggested that we drive Will to and from school rather than have him ride the bus. It wasn't an unreasonable idea. Having a seizure on the bus would not only be dangerous for Will but also for everyone else. Brian and I agreed it'd be for the best, so I've been driving him every day since.

The day after Halloween was no exception. I'd just picked the boys up from their respective school buildings, which happened to be across the street from each other, and had just started the short commute back home. Then, as we waited at the stop sign right outside of the school, our car was rocked to the side with a punishing jerk. We'd been crashed into by a bus. I couldn't believe it! Fortunately, the boys and I were all OK. The car, however, was not so lucky. My door had been smashed in so badly I couldn't even open it to get out. I had to crawl over the center console and get out through the passenger door. Then, I opened the rear passenger door and helped the kids get out. They were visibly shaken but thankfully unharmed. Their eyes were wide with disbelief as they took in the site of our crunched in car. To add to the spectacle, the wreck occurred at the busiest time of day. There were buses, cars, teachers, and students all over the place trying to get in and out of the school parking lot—all of them suddenly blocked by the accident clogging up the intersection.

As the chaos continued to bloom around us, I was happy and relieved to see a friendly face appear. My good friend Jodi was a couple of cars behind us when the accident occurred. After the kids and I got out of the car, she hopped out of hers to see if I needed help. The police had just arrived on the scene, and I knew it would probably be some time before everything got sorted out and I'd be free to go. So, when Jodi offered to take the boys with her to her house, I jumped on it, thanking her profusely for her steadfast kindness and generosity. We really do have the most amazing friends!

As soon as the boys were taken care of, I called Brian. He actually answered on the first ring, much to my surprise. He shocked me even more when he said, "I'll be right there." It was 3:30 in the afternoon and on a typical day he'd be at work nearly an hour away from home. My astonishment grew when a mere five minutes later I heard Brian's street-legal dirt bike as it roared up the hill. *No way!* I thought as he slowed to a stop right next to me. He was dressed in his full motorbike garb, complete with shin pads, riding boots, gloves, and helmet. Our neighbors had taken to calling him *Cool Rider* when they spotted him rocking his full racing gear. I was giving my statement to the nice officer when Brian arrived; it was comical!

Once he was certain that we were alright, he pulled his helmet back on and said, "I'll head home and grab my car."

"Good idea," I replied as I watched my car being lifted onto a flatbed tow truck.

I wasn't about to climb on the back of his motorbike to get home. Besides, we still had to go pick up the kids at Jodi's house. What a day! I couldn't get over the irony of it—to be hit by a school bus on school property while picking up my son who isn't allowed to ride the bus. I erupted in laughter at the thought of it all. Sometimes you just have to laugh at the curveballs life throws at you. You either laugh or you cry, right? So, I laughed to myself ... and it still makes me laugh to this day!

# CHAPTER 24
# WINNING

We'd had our fair share of challenges over the last year or two. Between the ups and downs of Will's epilepsy plus a broken arm, a concussion, earaches, and the bus collision, our little family of four really needed a break. With that in mind, I decided to cancel Will's pending adenoidectomy and ear tube surgery. I had no desire to put Will through one more test, let alone a surgical procedure at that time. The minor changes we'd made to his routine had helped ease the discomfort he'd been feeling so our sense of urgency had faded. I felt comfortable passing on the procedure and reevaluating whether to pursue it at a later date. Enough was enough! We needed to let off some steam and have a little fun.

Not long after Will went back on his anti-seizure meds, we started to see results. I couldn't believe how quickly his seizures diminished and how well he seemed to be feeling. In a matter of days, Will claimed they were gone, and I trusted his assessment. No one else on earth could be more in tune with Will's body and brain than himself.

With Will on the mend, we began to look for opportunities to have fun and relax. Will and Blake both decided to sign up to play recreational basketball—no traveling, no pressure— just fun. They were each assigned to teams by age and were disappointed to learn that none of their friends had been placed on either of their teams. Brian and I took the opportunity to explain to them both that, from here on out, they'd have to cope with being thrown into new situations with people they've never met, including teachers, coaches, teammates, and bosses. They needed to get over it, do the necessary work, and give their best for themselves and their teams.

As luck would have it, Blake's coach was spectacular. He had a vested interest in teaching these kids about the game and came to practice equipped with plays, diagrams, drills, and a positive attitude. Will had always been jealous of Blake's natural athletic ability and now he had reason to be jealous of Blake's coach and team. We tried our best to instill a work-hard mentality in them, but Will couldn't shake his resentment at how it just wasn't fair.

By the middle of the season, Blake's team was undefeated while Will's team was yet to win a single game. Blake's team always played before Will's, so each Saturday started with a *W* and ended with an *L*. It ruined the rest of the day for Will every single Saturday. He'd slog out of the gym deflated and depressed. To make matters worse, Will's coach had a ton going on in her personal life and seemed to bring it with her to the court. There was a lot of yelling and negativity, and the boys couldn't help but absorb it and spit it back out. They were disjointed and frustrated and took to blaming each other. They began putting each other down rather than trying to work together and cheering each other on. They were in a downward spiral that was twisting out of control. It was hard for the team and even harder to watch from the stands. Will wanted to quit, and we were saddened by it. This was supposed to be fun, a break from all the other drama that seemed to permeate our lives, but it had turned out to be anything other than fun. It felt like this horrible season would hang on forever.

Then my phone rang, and it was Will's coach. Her voice was hoarse, strained from the cold she'd been battling. It was Saturday morning, and the boys were packing their stuff up to head to the court. She asked if I would coach the team in her place. The game was happening in two hours! She thought she might be able to make it but just wasn't feeling up to the task. Although I had no prior basketball experience, I didn't want the boys to miss their game, and I felt up for the challenge. I knew, if nothing else, that I could bring my positive attitude to that gym and encourage those boys to have fun. I also hoped that my athletic husband might be able to help me out, but Brian had been called out to the hospital earlier that morning, and I wasn't sure if he'd be able to make it in time.

Before we left for the gym, I checked the schedule and realized Will's team was scheduled to play Blake's coach's other team. He had an older son who played as well and managed to somehow coach both teams. What are the odds? I really had my work cut out for me. He was going to show up prepared with plays and charts, and I didn't even know the names of my players yet, besides my own son.

When we arrived at the court, I saw a couple of girlfriends and explained the situation. I told them I might need to borrow one of their husbands when one of them looked at me confused and replied, "Why do you need my husband when your former Major League playing husband is right there?" Hallelujah! Brian made it! I was ecstatic when I saw him, so happy to have an assistant on the court. These boys needed a victory, and I was ready to do my best to make it happen.

We gathered the team at the bench and proceeded to review our plan for the game, which was to pretend they were playing a game of backyard basketball: no pressure, just fun. The other coach smiled and waved, clearly surprised to see Brian and I on the sidelines. It was ironic that I knew all his plays. I'd sat in the bleachers every week for Blake's practices and couldn't help but take note of the drills they practiced over and over again. Will was excited to tell his teammates that his mom knew the opposition's playbook, even though I had no intention of sharing any inside information.

I felt like this might be our chance to give Will a win and to leave that gym with a smiling son. We were determined, and the boys seemed to feed off our energy. We scored the first four points, and I was tempted to take a picture of the score board—proof positive that we'd had the lead. It was exhilarating, and the boys were on fire! They were passing the ball, communicating well on the court, and cheering each other on. After 40 fabulous minutes on the court, our team came out ahead. We got a *W!* The boys almost didn't know how to celebrate. They were in shock and so were we. Our debut as a coaching duo was a success, and Will was so happy. That win was the best win I have ever experienced in my life. Bigger than any win I witnessed my husband achieve in an MLB stadium, bigger than any all-star game of Blake's, and bigger than a Steeler's Super Bowl or Penguin's Stanley Cup game! This was a sign we'd won, and we would continue to win in our fight against epilepsy! Never give up, and whatever life deals you, just keep climbing.

# CHAPTER 25
# THE CLIMB

When I started writing this book over eight years ago (though it feels much longer than that to be honest), I was convinced that there would be some defining moment marking the end of Will's battle with epilepsy and therefore marking the end of this story. I imagined writing one final, heroic chapter celebrating our victory, wrapping it all up with a perfectly curled bow, and a stamp of good health. After our success with the ketogenic diet, I was convinced that we had won the battle against Will's seizures for good. The cruise was to be our ultimate victory lap as we sailed off into the sunset—literally and figuratively—and left all the terrifying and tumultuous days we'd somehow survived behind us.

Alas, life had other plans for us. It was a devastating turn of events when his seizures returned. A painful punch to the gut that left us reeling in shock and gasping for breath. Our perfect ending to Will's battle against the *bad guys* in his brain, and to this very book, had been completely ruined. We were devastated and angry. I honestly just didn't have it in me to continue telling Will's story for a very long time. Months went by before I could muster the strength to open my files and continue where I'd left off. We were still picking up the pieces of our broken hearts, still coming to grips with the undeniable fact that our fight wasn't over, and the lingering concern that it might never be.

But if Will's unpredictable struggle with epilepsy has taught me anything, it's been to count our blessings and live in the here and now. There is something to be grateful for every day when you take the time to think about it. For as rough as it has been for our family over the last several years, we've also been so fortunate. When I think of the countless families we've passed in the hallways at

Children's Hospital who were there with children much sicker than Will, I say a prayer and wish them strength. I also say a prayer of thanks that, while we'd spent many a night within those walls, we'd always been able to go home.

I used to scoff at the old adage, *What doesn't kill you makes you stronger*, but now I understand the sentiment behind it. We are all stronger, stauncher, and more determined than I ever imagined possible. Bolstered by our family's love and uplifted by the support of our friends and neighbors, we've found the courage to keep fighting, to keep climbing. We do our best to stay positive and maintain an attitude of gratitude. We relish the blissfully boring days we might otherwise take for granted. We dare to laugh, to dream, and to hope.

I know that probably sounds cliché like platitudes stolen from a worn-out motivational book, but we've chosen to embrace them. We cannot control what happens in life, but we can control how we react. We can choose to get back up when life knocks us down. We can choose to look for the good in even the worst of situations. We can choose to appreciate the things we have and to work hard for things that we want. We can choose to believe that there are better days ahead, not only for Will, but for all of us.

Will's story isn't over, far from it. As I write the final chapter of this book, he's now in seventh grade. His body and brain continue to grow, complete with a dizzying side of hormonal soup that's a typical part of the coming-of-age process. He's been, from what we can tell thus far, seizure-free since restarting this most recent course of medication and is feeling good. I'd like to say I'm confident that he'll stay that way and that his epilepsy has been cured. The realist in me recognizes that's not yet possible to predict.

Still, when I think about Will's future, I can't help but be optimistic. Even with all the trauma Will's brain has been through, it has never failed him. In fact, it's been downright blowing us away.

This compromised, overstimulated organ is helping Will score straight As in school, and we couldn't be any prouder. I think back to those grueling days when his cognitive development had been in question and the sleepless nights spent worrying about his ability to learn and grow, to become a functioning, contributing member of society. Isn't that the most basic desire parents have for their children? To be happy, healthy, independent, and useful? It's been such a relief to see him thrive in this regard and be able to put those fears to rest knowing, without a doubt, that Will can be that and so much more.

He has dreams, goals, and plans for the future. Now none of them feel out of reach. He wants to get a license and drive a car when he turns 16. He plans to graduate from high school and go off to college (and not have his mom for a roommate, thank you very much!). He dreams of becoming a doctor so that he might one day be able to help and heal others like so many doctors have helped him.

We love his dreams and will do anything we can to help make them come true! In the meantime, we'll continue to take one day at a time and do our best to keep him healthy. We *will* continue to believe, *Where there's a WILL, there's a way!*

# Epilogue
# Will's Way

After hearing a publisher leave a message on our answering machine the summer after Will's eighth-grade year, he came to me and asked me to not publish this book. "High school is going to be hard enough, and I don't need people to know about my disorder and my private life," he said.

There was no way I could go against his wishes; I needed to respect his privacy. After all, it was his battle and his story, so I needed his approval to share it with the world. His four years of high school proved to be challenging and not without drama. Thankfully, they were without seizures though! He remained basically healthy, played some basketball until injuries sidelined him, got a job, became a rated chess player, and continued to impress us academically—all with his brain disorder. He stayed on his anti-seizure medicine and continued to worry about not being able to get a driver's license.

After years of experience, we assumed that each and every appointment would be drama laden. Will hadn't been to Children's Hospital in over 700 hundred days, which was definitely a record for us. We thought it was important to be seen by a neurologist his senior year before leaving for college, so we decided to make it a proper outing with lunch included. His appointment wasn't until 2 p.m., so we headed out by 11:30 a.m. and hit a yummy sushi restaurant on our way. Will and I enjoyed a long leisurely lunch and covered topics from dating to going away to school. He has matured an incredible amount, and it is crazy to think he will be off on his own soon.

After paying our bill, we hopped in the car and made the drive downtown to the hospital. The sick-to-my-stomach nervous feeling filled my body as we entered the parking garage. The bad memories came to the surface as soon as we stepped in the elevator. The tests, multiple overnight stays, bloodwork, and stress of being in that hospital were front and center. I tried to block them out; I tried to focus on Will and how healthy he seemed ... and then we got to registration.

"Will Simmons?" she said twice.

I confirmed that was his name. While she typed away with a perplexed look on her face she replied, "You aren't in the system for today."

To which I responded, "Oh yes, we do have an appointment today. We have been emailed, called, and texted to remind us of this appointment."

After checking again, she said that we must have missed their call; the doctor that Will was supposed to see called off that day.

*Nope, not today!* I thought. I told her, "We have waited two years to see a doctor, and we are on a fieldtrip today. We will wait for the next available doctor." The receptionist was very kind, which was helpful. She said to give her a minute, and she would figure something out for us.

In the meantime, she asked, "What do you feed your child?" as she glanced at the six-foot-five teenager I had with me.

I responded, "Sushi. Today it was sushi."

Within ten minutes, we were being ushered down the hall to the neurology wing. First was a stop to get some vitals. Will's blood pressure was normal, but getting his height was not. The sweet, petit nurse couldn't reach the measuring lever to get it high enough for him! She said, "You must be the tallest boy in school!"

After weighing him, we were dropped off in the exam room. It seemed like forever until anyone came in. The door flew open, and a nursing student introduced herself. She said that she needed to get some information as she was doing a neurology rotation. I started to think we might not get to see a doctor after all.

Finally, after filling her in on Will's lengthy background, I politely asked, "Are we going to see a doctor today?" She said indeed we would, she just wasn't sure who as they were extremely shorthanded.

The next 20 minutes replay in my head over and over again. I was flabbergasted with how this *canceled* appointment transpired. In walked a young, handsome doctor with some pep in his step. I took note of and appreciated his very bright and positive entrance.

He sat down, checked Will's chart, and asked him, "Will, did you take your meds this morning?"

To which Will responded immediately, "Yes."

The next sentence out of the doctor's mouth rocked our world! He looked Will in the eye and delivered the best news we have ever heard.

He said, "Never take your morning meds again."

As tears started pouring out of my eyes, I said, "Can you repeat what you just said?"

Will was in shock, and I was fully crying. The sweet med student offered me a tissue and the doctor looked at Will and said, "Your mom has been worried about you for over a decade, these are tears of relief!" Man was he right!

This amazing human went on to give Will guidelines for weaning off his anti-seizure drug and tips on what to watch for along the way. I could sense that Will wanted to ask a question, and I pretty much knew what that question was ... *can I still drive?* So, to take the pressure off him, I asked the doctor if Will had any restrictions while weaning. He also knew what I was referring to and kindly looked at Will and asked him if he had his license. Will responded that he did.

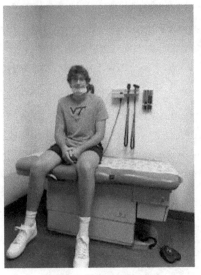

Our own Buddy the Elf

This amazing doctor said, "Just take it easy driving for a few weeks. Try not to drive long distances, (which he doesn't) and don't drive when you are tired. After two weeks, if you feel fine, resume normal driving practices."

The doctor was printing out what seemed to be an entire book.

After a couple minutes, I politely said, "May I ask what you are printing out?"

He said, "I am discharging Will today. He will no longer need to be a neurology patient here at Children's Hospital."

We began to feel like we had just won the lottery! Is this guy for real, and where has he been for the past 14 years? Will deserved this, and we worked hard for it. Now it was time to spread the good news!

I typically pulled out of that parking garage feeling defeated and discouraged, and often with new medications for Will to try or follow-up tests already scheduled. But this day was different—it was the best feeling in the world. For some strange reason, the gate lever was already lifted as we approached the exit. I knew it was a sign: no more barriers or hurdles to jump over. We were free! I laid on the gas and took the speed bump out of that garage like I was driving the General Lee in the *Duke's of Hazard!* We got air, looked at each other with tears in our eyes, and said *SEE YA!*

Life has not been a walk in the park for Will, but through it all, he has learned and gained so much. Often, the silver lining isn't clear until you are on the other side of whatever hardship you face. We faced his hardships together, and I wouldn't have it any other way. I will never forget the time Will caught me crying after he had a seizure. He asked what was wrong, and I explained to him that when he didn't feel well neither did I. After I spoke those words, I figured that was confusing for him. Nope! He said to me, "Wow, Mom, we are just like E.T. and Elliott!" He lived through some scary moments and would sometimes ask me some deep questions. "Are your eyes open in heaven?" "Is heaven a giant cloud?" and "How old is God?" It was almost as if his brain was focused on heaven, and it terrified me. These moments are engraved in my mind and heart, and I am happy to store them there and celebrate the good health he has been blessed with today.

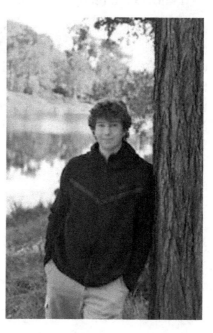

Will's senior photo

Will is headed off to college in the fall of 2023 to the University of Tennessee as a finance major. Rocky Top will become his new home sweet home!

We are overwhelmed with pride in all that he has accomplished. He is resilient and strong, and we know he is on the right path. Will finally gave me the green light to call the publisher back. He said he was ready to help others and wants kids who are facing tough diagnoses to find hope in his story. Will is no longer embarrassed about his journey. He is content in his own skin and ready to move on.

I know I am ready to move on as well.

This book has been many years in the making. It has served as my coping mechanism, so thank you for coming on this journey with us. We have been blessed with the most wonderful family, friends, and neighbors. Your love and support are appreciated more than you will ever know. We are here for you whenever you need us! And when life seems impossible, never forget, "Where there is a *WILL* there's a way!"

# Resources

We have created a Facebook page, called "A Mom's Will," for people to share stories, ask questions, and follow our journey. You can visit us at the link below:

www.Facebook.com/AMomsWill

## Helpful Websites

Doose Syndrome Epilepsy Alliance | Joining Forces to Create Change (https://doosesyndrome.org)

EAWCP - Epilepsy Association of Western and Central PA (https://eawcp.org)

Epilepsy Alliance America | Epilepsy Alliance Florida : Epilepsy Alliance Florida (https://epilepsyalliancefl.org/epilepsy-alliance-america)

How to Get Started With the Ketogenic Diet (charliefoundation.org)

Home - Matthew's Friends - Ketogenic Diet (matthewsfriends.org)

Epilepsy Foundation, #1 trusted site for epilepsy and seizure news (https://epilepsy.com)

Johns Hopkins Medicine, based in Baltimore, Maryland (https://hopkinsmedicine.org)

## Helpful Apps

Keto Calculator

Keto Diet

Keto Manager

Seizure Alert

## Helpful Books

*Ketogenic Diet Therapies for Epilepsy and Other Conditions,* Eric Kossoff, MD; Zahava Turner, RD, CSP, LDN; Mackenzie C. Cervenka, MD; and Bobbie J. Barron, RD, LDN

Epilepsy Journal for Children: Keep A Log of Your Child's Seizures, Medications, Triggers & Side Effects, Medjournal Essentials

Keto Kid: Helping Your Child Succeed on the Ketogenic Diet, Deborah Ann Snyder, DO

*The Ketogenic Diet Cookbook: Developed by the Ketogenic Diet Team at Children's Hospital of Philadelphia,* Christina Bergqvist, MD; Paige Vondran; Claire Chee; Meghan Walker; Sue Groveman; and Cagla Fenton

Parent's Guide to Using the Ketogenic Diet (Downloadable PDF), Charliefoundation.org

# THE EPILEPSY ASSOCIATION WALK
## WILL'S WARRIORS

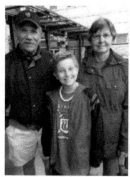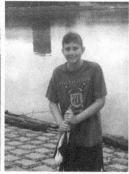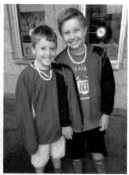

Will proudly with G-Daddy and Grandma (left), Our warrior, Will (center), Will and his buddy, Jack (right)

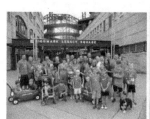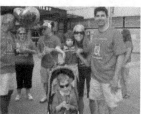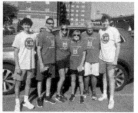

Will's Warriors team photo (left), Will taking a ride for a walk! (center), Grown-up Will with his parents, brother, Nonny, and Poppy (right)

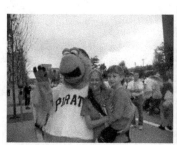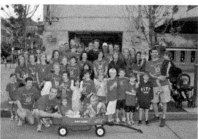

Pirate Parrot time! (left) Will's Warriors Inaugural Epilepsy Association Walk (right)

# SPECIAL THANKS

Special thanks to Janene Jost, my dear friend and talented "story guide" and developmental editor. Janene graduated with a degree in English literature and an MBA in marketing and human resources. She is an avid writer of all things from corporate content to creative fiction. Besides being super talented, she is a fabulous friend. Janene lived through each page of this book in real time and generously offered to relive it with me on paper. Her input, advice, and guidance during this process and over the years has been priceless. I am so proud to have her involved in this project, but I am even more proud to call her a friend. Thank you for always being there for us; your friendship means the world to me.

Special thanks to Andrew Jobling, teacher of "One Word at A Time" writing workshop. I took a chance on a virtual writing class ten years ago to see if I could possibly put Will's story on paper. Andrew taught, mentored, and motivated me all the way from Australia! My progression was often interrupted by months of medical leave so I could take care of Will, and Andrew continued to support my efforts for years. I am so proud to say I completed the course! The manuscript was the final step, and ten years later, here we are! Thank you, Andrew Jobling (retired professional Australian football player, best-selling author of eight books, and motivational speaker) for sharing your expertise and sticking with me!

Special thanks to Dr. Karen Orr, my doctor, friend, and foreword writer. I appreciate you and everything you have done for my family. I don't think you ever realized how instrumental you were in our healing. God definitely put us together.

And finally, thank you to my husband, Brian, for being by my side through it all. I am so glad you asked me to the homecoming dance so many years ago!

# About the Author

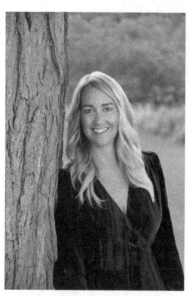

Details Photography by Melissa Novak

Jennifer Drake Simmons is a devoted mom to sons Will and Blake and wife to her high school sweetheart, Brian. She graduated with honors from Virginia Tech where she received a B.S. in nutrition and exercise science. Jennifer pursued a career in event planning and fundraising with The Leukemia & Lymphoma Society in Washington D.C. before she moved home to Pittsburgh, Penn.

Today, she stays busy making jewelry and volunteering on multiple boards and with booster clubs. Jennifer offers support, encouragement, and resources to families living with epilepsy.

CPSIA information can be obtained
at www.ICGtesting.com
Printed in the USA
JSHW011110140723
44601JS00002B/10